Prostate Cancer

A CLEVELAND CLINIC GUIDE

Eric A. Klein, M.D.

Cleveland Clinic Press

Cleveland, Ohio

Prostate Cancer

A CLEVELAND CLINIC GUIDE

Contact:
Cleveland Clinic Press
9500 Euclid Avenue NA32 / Cleveland, Ohio 44195
216-445-5547 / delongk@ccf.org
www.clevelandclinicpress.org

This book is not intended to replace personal medical care and supervision. There is no substitute for the experience and information that your doctor can provide. Rather, it is our hope that this book will provide additional information to help people understand the nature, diagnosis, and treatment of prostate cancer.

Proper medical care always should be tailored to the individual patient. If you read something in this book that seems to conflict with your doctor's instructions, contact your doctor. Since each case is different, there may be good reasons for individual treatment to differ from the information presented in this book. If you have any questions about any treatment in this book, consult your doctor.

The patient names and cases used in this book are composites drawn from several sources.

Library of Congress Cataloging-in-Publication Data

Klein, Eric A., 1955-
Prostate cancer : a Cleveland Clinic guide / Eric A. Klein.
p. cm.

Includes index.

ISBN 978-1-59624-086-5 (alk. paper)

1. Prostate – Cancer – Popular works. I. Title.

RC280.P7K538 2007   616.99′463 – dc22   2007029233

Cover and book design: J. Michael Myers
Medical illustrations: Joseph A. Pangrace, C.M.I.,
Cleveland Clinic Center for Medical Art and Photography

CONTENTS

Dedication

To prostate cancer patients everywhere,
who face difficult decisions with
hope and courage every day

Introduction

You have picked up this book because you have a reason for wanting to read about prostate cancer.

Type "prostate cancer" into a search engine on your computer and you will get more than 9.8 million hits. Some of the sites provide legitimate and useful information. Some provide information so technical and detailed that even molecular biologists will be forced to pause. Other sites promise cures developed from a magic powder made from tree roots found on the western slopes of the Himalayan Mountains and kept secret by monks for centuries.

Prostate cancer is a serious disease. In this book, which I have endeavored to make as readable as possible, I will present as much information about it as I can. I'll tell you as much as possible about prostate cancer, who gets it, how it is found, and how it is treated. But this text *should not* be your sole source of information. I advise you to read it with pen and paper at hand, so that you can write down questions and observations as they occur to you.

If you really want to find out about prostate cancer, the best way to do it is in a conversation with your doctor. He or she will advise you about the disease and, more important, answer questions as they apply to you or to a loved one who is undergoing treatment. Your job is to come up with the right questions. And that is where this book comes in.

A fellow named Dave will also help. You will meet him on the next page ...

Chapter 1

Who Gets
Prostate Cancer?

Dave does not know it yet, but he has prostate cancer.

Like most men in their late 50s, Dave is not even thinking about prostate cancer. Why should he? He knows that he is not in perfect shape now – he could get a little more exercise, drop a few pounds, cut back on the red meat – and he intends to take better care of himself. He even bought an exercise bike.

Dave would not even be sitting in the waiting room were it not for his wife, who has been urging him to get a checkup ever since her brother had coronary artery surgery last year. So Dave is now sitting on a vinyl couch skimming through an issue of *National Geographic.* Instead of thinking about prostate cancer, Dave is wondering what it would be like to stumble across ancient Aztec ruins like the ones depicted in the magazine lying open in his lap.

What Dave does not realize is that he is about to embark on another adventure altogether.

Dave is going to join an estimated 234,460 men who will be diagnosed with prostate cancer this year. But consider this: The U.S. Census Bureau estimates that there were about 61.9 million men age 50 and older in the United States in 2003. Therefore, slightly less than 0.4 percent of all the men of age 50 and older in the United States will be diagnosed with the cancer.

But this figure is somewhat misleading, because it represents only those men whose prostate cancer has been diagnosed. Statistically, there are many men in this age group who, like Dave, have prostate cancer and do not know it. According to the National Cancer Institute, all men have a 17 percent chance of developing the disease, and a man's risk of dying of prostate cancer is around 3 percent. This death rate reflects both the advances medicine has made during the past 50 years and the character of the disease.

Of all the cancers that beset men, prostate cancer is the most common and, when detected early, the most treatable. The five-year, cancer-specific survival rate for men with newly diagnosed disease is 100 percent. The 10-year survival in these same men is 92 percent. Compare these statistics to those for lung cancer, which has an overall five-year survival rate of less than 15 percent.

The prostate cancer death rate also says something about the nature of the cancer. It is a slow-growing cancer and many men, particularly those who acquire the disease later in life, are likely to die of causes other than the cancer.

All statistics are generalities, and care should be taken in their interpretation. There are different incidence rates among age groups, among nationalities, and even among geographic regions. For instance, the incidence of prostate cancer is higher in the United States than in China. This may be interpreted to mean that the cancer appears more frequently here than in China, or it may mean that it shows up more often in the United States because our doctors are more aggressive in looking for it.

In fact, the higher rate is a combination of both factors. When use of the prostate specific antigen (PSA) test became widespread in the early 1990s, the incidence of the cancer rose sharply. There was no sudden outbreak of the disease – the incidence increased because the new screening test allowed doctors to become more efficient at finding a disease that was already there. (You will learn more about PSA beginning with Chapter 3.)

On the other hand, Chinese men actually do have a lower risk of developing the cancer. This observation may mean that Chinese men have something in their genes that renders them less susceptible to the disease, or that there is something in their diet or in their lifestyle. Most epidemiologists – the men and women who study diseases as they affect societies and cultures – are inclined to believe that diet has something to do with the lower risk. Research on diet and nutrition seems to back this up. (We'll look at dietary substances thought to reduce the risk of prostate cancer in Chapter 7.)

RISK FACTORS

One of the great values of epidemiological data is that it can be translated into risk factors. American men have a higher incidence of prostate cancer than any other nationality. The incidence of the cancer among American men of all races is 173.8 detections per 100,000 men, as compared to 8.6 per 100,000 men in China.

Here is how other countries measure up to the U.S. rate (again, these international incidence rates are per 100,000 men):

United States	173.8	Denmark	29.9
Australia (New South Wales)	90.1	Poland (Warsaw)	22.2
Canada	80.2	Singapore	13.9
Sweden	63.0	Japan (Osaka prefecture)	9.0
Colombia, Chile	42.2	China (Hong Kong)	8.6
United Kingdom (England)	39.6	India (Mumbai)	7.4
Czech Republic	32.0		

Adapted from "Cancer Incidence on Five Continents," Vol. VIII, Lyon IARC, 2002. Edited by DM Parkin, SL Whelan, J Ferlay, L. Teppo and DB Thomas. *IARC Scientific Publication* No. 155, Lyon 2002; Surveillance and Risk Assessment Division, CCDPC Health Canada; http://www.cancer.ca/ccs/internet/standard/0,3182,3543_367655_379099032_langId-en,00.html.

This should be understood about risk factors: They are categorical comparative values. The statistics do not state Dave's chances of acquiring the disease; they just indicate the chances that men in his age category (American men in their late 50s) will be diagnosed with the cancer compared to the chances of men in another category (Chinese men in their late 50s).

Risk factors are generalities. A man may exhibit every known risk factor and live disease-free until he is 100 years old or more. Risk factors should be seen as flags, the medical equivalent of a Post-It™ note reminder to tell a man he should pay a little more attention to what is going on with his body.

These are the risk factors:

Age

At age 50, every U.S. male gets one of these Post-It™ note reminders. The risk for prostate cancer is not high now. Around 2 percent of all prostate cancers are diagnosed in men between the ages of 50 and 54. But this percentage climbs steadily as the years pass. Around 20 percent of all prostate cancer is found in men ages 65 to 69. Autopsies have found that 75 percent of men age 75 or older have microscopic evidence of prostate cancer.

There is another reason to be alert to age-related risks. Prostate cancer is slow-growing and is often without symptoms. But the good news is that the earlier the cancer is found, the more likely it is that treatment will lead to a favorable outcome. Notice in the chart on page 5 how the incidence of prostate cancer rises as men age.

Race

That Dave is a white male is worth noting because there are major differences among the races in terms of cancer risks and cancer deaths. Prostate cancer is the most common cancer in African Americans and the second leading cause of cancer-related deaths. (Lung cancer is the first; in fact, lung cancer is the leading cause of cancer-related deaths in Caucasians, also.) The American Cancer Society estimated that 30,770 African Americans had prostate cancer in 2005 and that another 5,050 men died of the disease that year.

Between 1997 and 2001 the incidence of prostate cancer was almost 60 percent higher in African Americans than in Caucasians. This means that 272.1 of every 100,000 African Americans were diagnosed with the cancer, compared to 164.3 of 100,000 Caucasians.

(Continued on page 6)

AGE AND PROSTATE CANCERS

Age	Percent of all prostate cancers diagnosed
Under 44 years	0.1 %
49	0.645 %
54	2.350 %
59	6.055 %
64	12.660 %
69	20.265 %
74	22.770 %
79	18.375 %
84	10.980 %
85 years and older	6.3 %

Source: J.L. Stanford, R.A. Stephenson, L.M.Coyle, et al. *Prostate Cancer Trends 1973-1995*, SEER Program, National Cancer Institute. NIH Pub. No. 99-4543. Bethesda, MD, 1999.

Prostate Cancer Comparisons by Race

According to the U.S. National Institutes of Health, for black men the incidence rate is about 60 percent higher than it is for white men and the mortality rate is about twice as high. The American Cancer Society makes the following comparisons:

- Incidence for prostate cancer among African Americans is 272.1 per 100,000 population, compared to 164.1 for Caucasians.
- Mortality among African Americans is 73.0, compared to 30.2 for Caucasians.
- Lifetime risk of the disease among African Americans is 20.6 percent, compared to 17.6 percent for Caucasians.
- Lifetime risk of death from the disease is 4.7 percent among African Americans, compared to 2.8 percent for Caucasians.

An even grimmer finding indicates that African Americans are more than twice as likely to die of the disease as Caucasians are.

These differences are significant, but the causes of the differences are unknown. Speculation centers around differences in genetic makeup, differences in the way tumors originate and grow, diet, lifestyle, average body mass, testosterone levels, health-care system bias, cultural attitudes toward health care, and various combinations of all the above factors.

Other numbers suggest that the differences may not be as great as many had thought initially. The incidence of "organ-confined disease" (cancer in its earliest stage, before it has spread beyond the prostate) at diagnosis is increasing and the disparity in death rates is declining. The two statistics are related. When the cancer is diagnosed and treated at the organ-confined stage, the five-year survival rate is 100 percent, regardless of race. So, if ever there were an argument for taking the screening test for prostate cancer, this is it.

Another question is this: Because the cancer in these men may behave differently, should the "scores" they receive on screening tests be evaluated differently? As of this writing, research has not revealed a simple answer to this question.

There are differences between races beyond those of African Americans and Caucasians. The age-adjusted annual rate of prostate cancer among American Indians and Alaskan natives is 50 cases per 100,000. Among Asians and Pacific Islanders it is 105 per 100,000, and for Hispanics it is 140 per 100,000. Are genes involved? Perhaps, but the more likely explanation lies with lifestyle and diet. This is good news because genes are steadfast in families, but lifestyle and diet can be changed. Those aspects of lifestyle and diet that may prevent prostate cancer are discussed in Chapter 7.

Genes

Cancer develops when one or more of the genes that control a cell's reproduction and growth go awry. Sometimes these genes are passed down through generations as an inheritance; sometimes they are disrupted by contact with compounds in the environment such as those found in nicotine; and sometimes they go awry for reasons that have yet to be found. One of the newest theories is that rogue cells are *always* present in the body, and when our immune system breaks down for some reason, the rogue cells become cancerous and begin to proliferate.

Whatever the case, a man with prostate cancer in his family history is at increased risk of developing the disease. The risk increases with the number of affected relatives, how closely related they are, and the man's age at diagnosis. For example, a man with a father or brother diagnosed with prostate cancer is twice as likely to be diagnosed with the cancer as a man who has no such cancer in his immediate family.

So if Dave has three brothers who have been diagnosed with the cancer, his risk is greater than if only one of the three brothers is diagnosed. And the age at which Dave's father or brothers are diagnosed may also be a factor. In addition, the younger his father or brothers were when they were diagnosed, the greater the risk of his being diagnosed with the cancer.

Here's how the risk percentage works out with family groups. (Bear in mind that first-degree relative equals father, brother, and son; second-degree relative equals grandfather, uncle, and nephew.)

- Any second-degree relative with prostate cancer (PCa) at any age   1.7
- Father with PCa   2.2
- A first-degree relative diagnosed with PCa after age 65   2.4
- Any first-degree relative with PCa at any age   2.6
- A first-degree relative diagnosed with PCa before age 60   3.3
- Brother with PCa   3.4
- Two or more first-degree relatives diagnosed at any age 5.1

Adapted from Aeegers MP, Jellema A, Ostrer H. "Empiric risk of prostate carcinoma for relatives of patients with prostate carcinoma: a meta-analysis." *Cancer* 2003;97:1894-1903.

Other Risks

A host of other factors have been associated with an increased risk of prostate cancer. While many of these risk associations are speculation, they bear mentioning as intriguing ideas to keep in mind.

Sexually transmitted diseases. Infection with one or more sexually transmitted diseases appears to raise the relative risk of prostate cancer. The risk varies according to the disease. A man with a history of any STD has a relative risk for prostate cancer of 1.44. If the disease is gonorrhea, the relative risk is 1.34. If the disease is syphilis, the relative risk is 2.30. Prostatitis, an inflammation of the prostate, raises the relative risk for prostate cancer to 1.57.

Vasectomy. A survey of medical studies of men with vasectomies suggests that the procedure might raise the risk of prostate cancer in these men to 1.37. However, it also may be that prostate cancer was found in these men because they were more likely to have been seen by a urologist. Urologists are particularly sensitive to prostate cancer.

This is also an example of how easy it can be to overlook epidemiological factors (such as what type of physician a man consults and how often he visits that doctor) as well as how scientific observation can turn into urban legend ("vasectomies cause cancer"). In other words, the relationship between vasectomies and prostate cancer is unknown – if one exists at all.

Smoking. Cadmium is one of a hundred toxins in cigarette smoke. The heavy metal is known to affect hormone levels and put cells under significant stress. The link between smoking and prostate cancer is tenuous, but the link between smoking and lung cancer is definite. If you are diagnosed with lung cancer, chances are good that you will not be around long enough to worry about your prostate.

Diet. The role that diet plays in increasing or decreasing the risk of prostate cancer comes from migration and immigration studies. Asians have the lowest incidence of prostate cancer in the world. However, when men from China, Japan, and other Asian nations move to the United States, the incidence of prostate cancer in their children rises significantly. There are several possible explanations

for why this happens, including change in diet, environmental exposure, and exposure to new infectious agents.

The relationship of diet to prostate cancer and a host of other cancers
is being intensively studied for two reasons. Identifying substances in
diets that create risks allows those substances to be eliminated.
Second, there may also be a number of substances that confer a
degree of protection. For example, foods such as blueberries are
reputedly high in antioxidants, and many herbalists believe that
drinking tea made from saw palmetto will naturally protect the
prostate. Those foods and natural substances that appear to confer a
degree of protection will be noted in Chapter 7.

Alcohol. The relationship between alcohol and prostate cancer is
not known, but many experts think it is similar to the relationship
between alcohol and heart disease – a little is good, but a lot is not.
Several studies have shown that a daily glass or two of red wine can
be healthy, presumably because of the antioxidant activity of the
polyphenolic compounds in the wine. At least one study has shown
that consumption of one to four glasses of red wine a week will
reduce the risk of prostate cancer.

This chapter began with the question: Who gets prostate cancer?
The answer is that just about all men will get it, if they live long
enough. A more appropriate question is *when* do men get prostate
cancer? In response to that question, most doctors would suggest that
starting around age 50, it is time to start paying attention to your
prostate health. If you are African American or have a father or brother
with the disease, you should probably start paying attention to these
risks a little earlier in life, around age 45. Staying aware of these risks
is not difficult or time-consuming. The standard screening tests for
prostate cancer are the digital rectal examination and the prostate
specific antigen (PSA) test. We'll talk about those tests in just a bit,
but first let's look at the prostate itself. ◆

Chapter 2

What Is a Prostate?

The prostate gland is actually a collection of many smaller glands that are encased by a layer of fibrous tissue called the prostatic capsule, which is surrounded by a layer of fat. The prostate gland is divided into right and left lobes. The base of the prostate is closest to the bladder; the apex is farthest away.

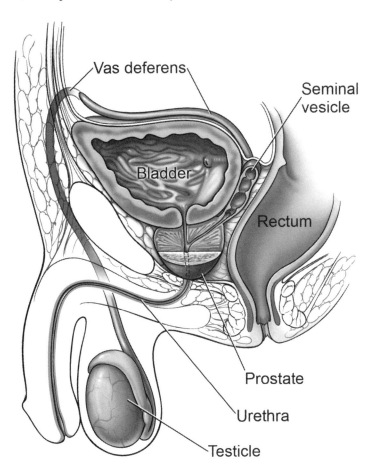

The prostate gland excretes a fluid that nourishes and protects sperm as it leaves the male urethra during the process of ejaculation. The gland's musculature (preprostatic tissue) encloses the urethra like a handshake and clasps it firmly during ejaculation, closing the urethra at one end while semen is being expelled from the other.

On a philosophical note, it might be observed that the prostate is more essential to the species than to the individual. Although a man can function perfectly well without the ability to reproduce efficiently, the same cannot be said of the species. In other words, a man can lose his prostate without it affecting the span of his years. However, the survival of our species would be severely challenged without the contributions made by the prostate.

Dave's prostate is average: a walnut-sized structure that wraps around the urethra just below the bladder. The prostate is an essential part of the male reproductive system, which includes the testes, the epididymis, the vas deferens, the seminal vesicles, and the prostate.

Sperm, created in the testes, is stored in the epididymis before traveling along the vas deferens en route to ejaculation. The seminal vesicle contributes mucus to the sperm, and the prostate adds a fluid containing calcium, zinc, citric acid, acid phosphatase, albumin, and prostate specific antigen (PSA). This slightly basic fluid gives the ejaculate its milky color. The fluid is necessary because the vagina's membranes and secretions create an acidic environment intended to discourage infectious microbes. Prostatic secretions bathe the sperm, nourish them, assist in lubricating the vagina, and provide a base that insulates sperm from the acidity found in the vagina. PSA and prostatic acid phosphatase are among numerous compounds found in the fluid. They will be referred to later in relation to detecting prostate cancer and as potential targets for treatment.

About 70 percent of the prostate is glandular. The remaining 30 percent is muscle. The gland comprises three zones: a peripheral zone, a transition zone (which surrounds the urethra), and a central zone. The functions of these zones are still being researched, but most prostate cancer occurs in the peripheral zone. In young adults, about 65 percent of the gland is peripheral zone tissue; 10 percent of the tissue lies in the transition zone, and 25 percent is in the central zone. Most prostate tumors (up to 90 percent) begin in the peripheral zone, and between 10 and 15 percent appear in the transition zone. The transition zone is also the area where benign prostatic hyperplasia occurs.

The nerves and vessels responsible for erections run along the flanks of the prostate "like racing stripes on a Chevy," as one expert put it. These nerves are an important consideration in prostate cancer treatments and will be further discussed in the therapy section (Chapter 5) of this book.

One of the characteristics of the prostate gland that sets it apart from others is that it has a unique growth pattern. The gland is formed during fetal development and grows to a weight of about 1.5 grams, the weight of about five paperclips. A second growth spurt begins during early puberty, when it grows to 11 grams as male hormones start circulating. The gland begins growing again when a man is in his early to mid-20s, reaching a weight of approximately 18 grams. The gland then remains stable for the next 30 years or so. When a man reaches his 50s, the gland again starts to grow and may reach a weight of 31 grams by the time he is 70.

One of the characteristics of the prostate gland that sets it apart from others is that it has a unique growth pattern.

However, many men have glands that exceed 50 grams, and some will reach more than 200 grams (almost half a pound). During this final growth spurt, the organ may become less of an asset and more of an impediment. This final growth is called "benign prostatic hyperplasia" (BPH). Although BPH is not life-threatening (hence the term benign), the growth of the gland can severely affect a man's quality of life. As it grows, it restricts the urethra and puts pressure on the bladder. This restriction limits a once powerful flow of urine to a trickle. The resultant pressure on the bladder gives rise to problems of urinary urgency and frequency. Urgency is the feeling that one has to urinate immediately, and frequency is when the feelings of urgency show up every hour or more. Although most prostate cancer is asymptomatic, similar symptoms can occur in some cases of prostate cancer.

There are medicinal and surgical solutions to BPH and other urological problems, many of which are associated with aging. Information on these problems is dependent on an accurate diagnosis, and an accurate diagnosis requires a visit to a urologist. But prostate cancer, which is much more dangerous, needs a different form of treatment. ◆

Chapter 3

How Is Prostate Cancer Found?

At age 50 (earlier for men with a family history of prostate cancer), you should have a routine physical that includes a discussion with your family physician, internist, or urologist on the pros and cons of a prostate cancer screening test.

There is a great deal of controversy surrounding this issue because no studies have shown that screening for prostate cancer using digital rectal examination (DRE) and prostate specific antigen (PSA) tests makes it less likely that a man will die from prostate cancer. However, there are good reasons to consider being screened.

Prostate tumors grow so slowly that they may be around for years before making their presence known, and most men exhibit no symptoms.

First, prostate tumors grow so slowly that they may be around for years before making their presence known, and most men exhibit no symptoms. Some may experience an odd sensation or pain in the region below their navels, which indicates that the cancer is present. But in most instances, the cancer hides quietly, and the only way it can be found is if someone goes looking for it.

Second, it is well established that the earlier the cancer is detected, the more likely that treatment will be successful, and it is well established now that PSA screening does result in earlier diagnosis.

Certainly, waiting for symptoms to appear is a bad idea. It is like waiting for your car engine to start making loud, unusual sounds before checking the oil.

If undetected, the cancer may grow to a point where it will begin to generate symptoms. These may include:

- Trouble urinating
- Frequent urges to urinate, especially at night
- Thin or weak urine stream
- Pain or burning when passing urine
- Pain or burning when ejaculating
- Blood in urine (hematuria)
- Blood in semen
- Nagging pain in the back, hips, or pelvis

Few men, if any, will feel *all* these symptoms. In fact, about 75 percent of men with advancing prostate cancer will experience none of these symptoms at all.

To further complicate matters, the aforementioned symptoms are associated with a host of diseases other than prostate cancer. Still, the value of symptoms is that they eventually become uncomfortable enough to send a man to a doctor.

Physicians want to catch the cancer before it begins to extend beyond the prostate. The first tool they use is an index finger. During a DRE, a physician probes a man's prostate by gently rubbing it with the tip of a finger inserted in the rectum. The ability to detect subtle differences in the size, shape, texture, and solidity of a prostate gland is as important a skill as picking up on a faint heart murmur or a soft wheeze in a patient's lungs.

The second initial test in the examination is the PSA (prostate specific antigen) test. It is important to understand at the outset that a PSA test, regardless of the findings, does not in any way constitute a diagnosis of prostate cancer. The test merely suggests whether further, more conclusive testing should be pursued. The test, introduced in the 1980s, detects a small protein (a glycoprotein), which is produced exclusively by prostatic epithelial cells. These cells might well be called "surface cells," because they line the surfaces of bodies and organs on both the outside and inside of cavities and chambers.

The physiological function of prostate specific antigen is to liquefy semen to make it easier for sperm to move about. The value of the PSA test lies not in its ability to detect the antigen in a blood sample, but in its ability to *quantify* the amount of the submicroscopic molecule present in a given volume of blood. As noted, the prostate expresses PSA as a fundamental component of semen, so finding PSA in a blood sample is common. Every man has some. The amount of PSA is what's important. The importance of specific amounts of PSA per milliliter (1/1000 of a liter, or 1/950th of a quart) has been the subject of discussions ever since the molecular assay was introduced.

THE PSA TEST

The debate over the merit of the PSA test revolves around three concepts of disease assays: sensitivity, specificity, and positive predictive value.

Sensitivity refers to a test's ability to identify a disease, not its ability to detect a molecule. The PSA test is exceedingly powerful at detecting the PSA molecule. It can present readings as low as 0.001 ng/mL PSA. Translated, that means there is 1/1000 of a nanogram of PSA for every milliliter of fluid. That is not much. A nanogram weighs a billion times less than one gram and almost a trillion times less than a pound. A milliliter is 1/1000 of a liter, about 950 times smaller than a quart.

The ability to detect such minuscule amounts of a molecule is not what medical professionals mean when they refer to a test's sensitivity. They are speaking of its ability to indicate the true presence of disease. If a cancer test or screen has a sensitivity of 70 to 80 percent, it means that the test will be positive for 70 to 80 of every 100 people with the cancer. The PSA assay has a sensitivity in the 70 to 80 percent range, but with some qualifiers. It only reaches this sensitivity for men who are 50 to 55 years old and have a PSA that is 4 ng/mL or higher. When the parameters change – when PSA levels fall below 4 ng/mL or rise substantially above that, or when the test is conducted in younger men or older men – the sensitivity changes.

Two landmark studies published in 2005 and 2006 sought to determine whether PSA was indeed the conclusive benchmark test that could tell men for sure whether or not they had prostate cancer. The study followed more than 18,000 men aged 55 or older over a seven-year period and used their PSA tests to predict their prostate health. Researchers found that:

- 15 percent of men with a PSA under 4 (the "normal" cutoff) had prostate cancer, and 15 percent of that group had high-grade cancers
- There is no PSA below which the risk of having cancer is zero (6.6 percent of men with a PSA of 0.5 have cancer)
- There is no true "normal" level of PSA, and decisions on biopsy need to be individualized based on absolute value of PSA, its rate of change over time, and other risk factors including DRE, family history, race, and prior biopsy results

And, after all that, what did the study prove? That PSA is a good but not perfect screening test.

Specificity refers to a test's ability to predict the absence of a disease when it isn't there. It is the proportion of nondiseased patients correctly identified by the test as not having the disease. The specificity of the PSA assay is 91 percent, which means that when the test indicates that cancer is not there, nine out of 10 times it is right.

Positive predictive value, the third testing concept, is the probability that a person will have the disease when the test says he should have the disease. The general positive predictive value of a PSA greater than 4.0 ng/mL in a man 50 or older is about 30 percent on biopsy. This means that when the test indicates that cancer might be present in one of these men and the doctor looks for it with a biopsy needle, he will find it one-third of the time.

The predictive value of PSA varies with its level. When the PSA falls into the "gray range" of 4.0 to 10.0 ng/mL, a biopsy will find cancer about 35 percent of the time. When PSA is above 10.0 ng/mL, a biopsy will find cancer about 50 percent of the time.

The problem is further complicated, because PSA is a fickle molecule – the production of which is affected by a host of factors. Benign prostatic hyperplasia (BPH, described in Chapter 2), prostatic inflammation (prostatitis), and perineal trauma or an injury to the region all can cause elevations in PSA levels. Not only does BPH alter PSA levels, but finasteride, the primary therapy for BPH, has been shown to affect PSA levels also, lowering them by half in the absence of cancer.

BPH is one of several conditions a physician must rule out when considering a diagnosis of prostate cancer. Prostatitis, an infection or inflammation of the prostate, is another. Symptoms of this condition include tenderness in the region and urgency, frequency, and a burning sensation when urinating. Again, these are symptoms similar to those created by prostate cancer.

PSA is also affected by diet, exercise such as bicycling, and trauma to the region. (For example, the hard grounder to second base that takes an unexpected and embarrassing hop at the last moment when you stoop to field it.)

The vagaries inherent in PSA testing are an important consideration and have been the subject of long and sometimes heated discussions in medical circles. It is worth restating: A PSA test *does not, cannot* diagnose prostate cancer. At best, the test indicates that further exploration is needed. This comes in the form of a biopsy, which is the only way to reliably secure a diagnosis. But the conflict stems from the fact that a biopsy is an invasive procedure that grates against a fundamental dictum of medicine: "First, do no harm." The conflict between the PSA screening test and a biopsy is that the PSA test generates a lot of false positives – up to 60 percent in some series of tests. This can translate into a great many unnecessary biopsies. Although there is little risk of complications associated with a prostate biopsy, it is not a completely innocuous procedure. Complications requiring hospitalization following the procedure are less than 1 percent, but up to half the men undergoing a prostate biopsy report pain and discomfort associated with the procedure.

Biopsies are good at finding cancers, but they do not necessarily distinguish what are termed "biologically significant" cancers from indolent ones. A biologically significant cancer is one that is certain to have an impact on an individual's health. An indolent tumor is one that is small and stable or is growing so slowly that it will never pose a health threat.

These subtle considerations can be lost on men like Dave and most people of either sex whose worst nightmares are conjured by the word "cancer." Of all the diseases that trouble humankind, cancer is the one that doctors hate the most. So when cancer is found, treatment usually follows, either on the advice of the doctor or at the insistence of the patient. When the tumor is indolent, chances that treatment will do more harm than good are substantial.

The challenge facing medicine is where to establish the "PSA cutoff." What level of PSA is likely to maximize the possibility of finding cancer on a biopsy while minimizing the number of biopsies conducted in men who do not have the cancer?

It might be possible to catch nearly every prostate cancer by lowering the PSA cutoff to something like 1.0 ng/mL. This means that physicians would be conducting biopsies on practically every middle-aged man who walked into their offices. They would be finding plenty of cancer. They would also be conducting plenty of unnecessary biopsies, finding many indolent cancers, and initiating a lot of unnecessary treatments.

Conversely, raising the PSA cutoff to 10 ng/mL would almost certainly ensure that every biopsy procedure would detect cancer. However, refraining from conducting any biopsies in men with PSA levels below 10 ng/mL means that many cancers would go undiagnosed and would progress. It must be noted again that catching a cancer early, while it is still confined to the prostate, vastly improves the success of any subsequent therapeutic procedures. Therefore, the decision to have a biopsy should be based on a discussion with your physician that includes consideration of known risk factors, including age, family history, race, DRE, and rate of change in PSA over prior determinations.

There have been refinements to the PSA assay that some feel render it a little more accurate. Correlating the PSA levels with the size of the prostate as measured by transrectal ultrasound (TRUS) can sometimes distinguish between cancer and BPH. Ultrasound might be said to be biological sonar. Under this procedure, completely harmless sound waves are emitted from a probe inserted into the rectum. The echoes of these waves as they bounce off organs and tissues of varying densities are analyzed by a computer to create images of the organs. Comparing the PSA levels with the size of the prostate may better reflect the increase in PSA levels associated with BPH.

Another way to distinguish cancer from BPH is to measure PSA velocity. PSA levels rise more rapidly in men with prostate cancer. To get a reliable indicator of velocity, a minimum of three tests should be given over a two-year period. This approach may have some utility in men whose antigen levels fall into the "gray area" of 4.0 to 10.0 ng/mL. One study found that a PSA velocity of 0.75 ng/mL a year was able to distinguish prostate cancer from BPH about 90 percent of the time. The drawback to PSA velocity is that it can take up to two years to get an accurate reading and, if cancer is present, it will be growing.

Free versus total PSA (f/t PSA) and complexed PSA (cPSA) are more refinements to the standard PSA. These assays compare differing types of PSA to enhance the specificity and sensitivity of the standard test. A certain amount of PSA is bound up with other proteins while other PSA remains free in the blood serum. Comparing the amount of free PSA to the amount of total (free plus bound) PSA gives a ratio that may help in making diagnostic decisions in men whose PSA falls into that troublesome gray range of 4.0 to 10.0 ng/mL.

For instance, Dave's PSA is 5.8 ng/mL and he has no symptoms. Under these circumstances, there is a 70 to 80 percent chance that a biopsy will turn up the cancer. To make both Dave and his physician feel a little better about deciding to conduct a biopsy, Dave's PSA levels are analyzed again, this time with a free-versus-total assay. The results show that of all the PSA in Dave's blood serum, 10 percent of it is free PSA. At this level, there is a 95 percent chance that when the physician goes looking for prostate cancer with a biopsy needle, it will be found.

BIOPSY

A biopsy – prostatic or otherwise – is a procedure in which a sample of tissue is obtained for study. The procedure requires that Dave do a bit of preparation. Men scheduled for the procedure are asked to avoid taking aspirin for five to seven days before the procedure. Aspirin is a blood-thinner, and avoiding its use will minimize the risk of bleeding. Men are also asked to stop taking anti-inflammatory drugs such as ibuprofen, Motrin, Advil, and others about three days before the procedure. A brief course of antibiotics is initiated a day or two before the biopsy, and Dave may be asked to take an enema to remove feces and gas from the rectum.

There are two primary instruments used in a prostate biopsy: a high-frequency ultrasound probe and a spring-loaded biopsy gun, neither of which is as ominous as its name would imply. The probe is

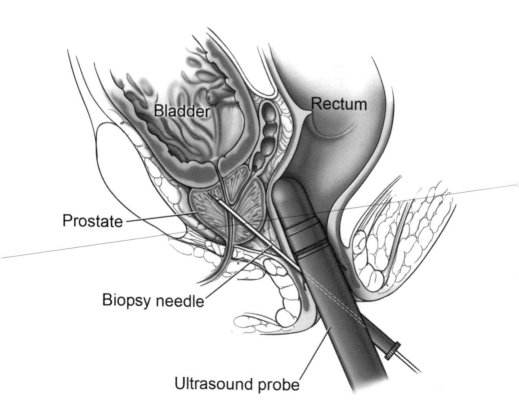

a slender tube, and the frequency of the sound waves is such that they are physically undetectable. The only way to know that the instrument is turned on is to look at the control board and its accompanying screen.

The biopsy gun is a cylinder holding a spring-driven needle. There is not much tissue separating the prostate from the wall of the rectum. The image produced by the TRUS technology allows the doctor to place the needle housing in the rectum, target the appropriate area of the prostate, and pull the trigger. The tiny biopsy needle, about 1.2 millimeters in diameter and less than half an inch long, enters the prostate, acquires a core sample of tissue, and returns to its sheath in a fraction of a second. Usually, a local anesthetic is injected around the prostate to help numb the sensation prior to the biopsy.

The physician will take a minimum of six tissue samples and probably more. Several studies have shown that increasing the number of tissue samples increases the likelihood that one of the samples will contain tissue from the cancer, if it is there. If all tissue samples prove negative – if they contain no cancerous tissue, but the patient's PSA levels remain inexplicably high – a repeat biopsy might be called for. An initial biopsy, even one taking eight samples, has a 5 to 15 percent chance of missing a cancer.

The tissue samples are sent to a pathologist, a specialist who studies the way diseases affect cells. The pathologist's report on the state of the cells in the sample will be combined with all other clinical information gathered, the DRE, PSA levels, and symptoms if present, to make a diagnosis. In Dave's case, depending upon what the pathologist does or does not find, Dave and his physician may have a long, serious talk. ◆

Chapter 4

Getting a Picture of Prostate Cancer

No two cancers have the same character.

In light of this fact, the next step for the physician treating Dave's prostate cancer is to learn as much as possible about the cancer's extent and nature. The characteristics of the tumor that emerge from ensuing diagnostic studies will help Dave and his doctor to determine one of several courses of therapy. Many treatment options are available, ranging from a variety of surgical procedures to an equal number of radiation and hormonal treatments.

The characteristics of the tumor that emerge from ensuing diagnostic studies will help Dave and his doctor to determine one of several courses of therapy.

The goal of the team of specialists now gathering around Dave's case is to get the best possible description of the cancer in order to narrow the treatments down to those that will be the most effective, yet engender the least trauma. It is no more necessary to shoot a fly with an elephant gun than is it appropriate to whack an elephant with a flyswatter.

There are essentially four aspects of Dave's clinical situation that need to be characterized in as much detail as possible before a course of therapy can be considered. These are:

- Dave's age and general health
- The amount of PSA being produced by his prostate
- The character or nature of the cancer cells in the tumor
- The extent of the tumor

HEALTH AND AGE

For Dave, who is in his late 50s, this may not be a problem. Many, perhaps most, prostate cancers grow slowly and do not become life-threatening for years. If Dave were in his mid- to late 70s, the chances are good that he would die of causes other than the cancer, especially if he had other health problems and the cancer were suspected to be small. Dave's age and other conditions are not deciding considerations, but they are aspects of his personal history that will be factored into an equation that will help determine a course of therapy. The principle is that if surgery or radiation therapy is not going to extend life, the procedures probably should not be employed because they can have an impact on quality of life.

PSA LEVELS: THE SHADOW OF THE BEAST

As noted in the preceding chapter, PSA levels help determine whether a diagnosis of prostate cancer should be pursued. PSA also helps fill in the emerging picture of the cancer. These levels do not present an exact picture; they are more like the "shadow" the tumor casts, but that shadow holds useful information.

Dave's "shadow," or PSA, is good news for him and his wife: 5.8 ng/mL is considered promising. That is, men with PSA levels between 4.0 ng/mL and 10.0 ng/mL have a 70 to 80 percent chance that the tumor will be confined to the prostate. Physicians call this "organ-confined" disease, and it is the most curable form of the disease.

PSA levels are also related to the likelihood that a prostate cancer may return after treatment. While PSA levels do not predict whether a cancer will recur, the higher the PSA , the higher the risk of recurrence. One study of more than 1,600 men with the same character of prostate cancer found that 81 percent of those with PSA levels below 10 ng/mL remained free of evidence of the disease for five years following radiation therapy.

HISTOPATHOLOGY: A CLOSER LOOK

The tissue acquired by biopsy is sent to a pathologist – a histopathologist, to be specific – who is familiar with the normal and abnormal characteristics of cells. The pathologist will peer at the cells in the tissue samples and assign them two Gleason scores: one for the character of the majority of diseased glands he spots and a second score for the remainder.

Gleason scores are named for Dr. Donald F. Gleason, who developed a system for judging the aggressiveness of a prostate cancer. Basically, when a pathologist looks at a prostate cancer specimen under the microscope, he will identify two architectural patterns – a primary or most common pattern and a secondary or second most common pattern – and assign a grade to each one. Glands are graded from 1 to 5, and scores are determined primarily by how much the appearance of an individual microscopic gland differs from normal. For example, a score of 1 indicates that *all* glands are relatively well defined and close to normal. A score of 5 indicates glands with boundaries that are very poorly defined. These glands are growing with no constraints. In other words, a Gleason grade 5 indicates a highly aggressive or rapidly growing tumor.

Gleason reasoned that by combining the grades of the two most common patterns he found in a patient's specimens, he could predict the likelihood that that particular patient would fare well or poorly.

Gleason reasoned that by combining the grades of the two most common patterns he found in a patient's specimens, he could predict the likelihood that that particular patient would fare well or poorly. The Gleason score that a physician gives to a patient is a combination of two numbers, which can be determined as follows:

- The best possible Gleason score, 2 (1 + 1), occurs when both the primary and secondary patterns have a Gleason grade of 1. However, most pathologists no longer consider any tumor with a Gleason score lower than 6 to be cancerous.

- The most common Gleason scores are 6 and 7; these are composed of patterns 3 + 3 for Gleason 6 tumors and either 3 + 4 or 4 + 3 for Gleason 7 tumors.

- The worst possible Gleason scores are 8 and above (4 + 4, 4 + 5, 5 + 5), when the primary and secondary patterns both indicate the presence of an aggressive tumor.

Here's how the test works in Dave's case: Most of the glands in Dave's tumor are mildly differentiated (Gleason grade 3), but there are some that are a little more distorted (grade 4). Dave's tissue samples are given a score of Gleason 3 + 4, which adds up to a Gleason score

How is the Gleason Score Calculated?

Prostate cancer growth patterns, as seen through a microscope (below left). In most cases, a pathologist can identify two architectural patterns – one primary or most common and one secondary or second most common. Both are graded in aggressiveness from 1 to 5. The final Gleason score is the sum of the two grades.

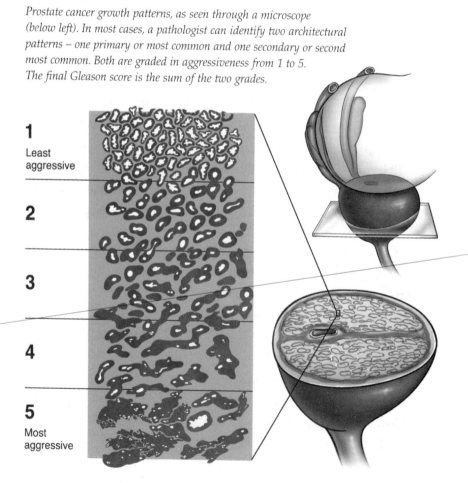

1
Least
aggressive

2

3

4

5
Most
aggressive

of 7, so Dave's tumor is considered to be an intermediate grade entity. Scores of 6 are known as low grade, 7 as intermediate grade, and 8 to 10 are high grade.

Gleason tumors with a total score of 6 or 7 account for about 90 percent of all prostate cancers. Gleason sum 7 tumors can be 3 + 4 or 4 + 3, depending upon which glandular pattern is predominant. Unlike the results of grade-school arithmetic, in prostate cancer 3 + 4 does not equal 4 + 3. The reason is that the aggressiveness of the tumor is determined by the amount of the highest-scoring tumor, so that a tumor that is 4 + 3 generally behaves more aggressively than a tumor that is 3 + 4, even though the sum for each is 7.

STAGING

PSA is said to be the shadow of the cancer. Pathology describes the cancer's character and determines its degree of aggressiveness. Staging completes the picture; it describes the cancer's extent and its physical presence.

There are two types of staging: clinical and pathologic. In clinical staging, specialists use all their experience and every tool available that will help them describe the size of a tumor or tumors and the extent or spread of the cancer. In pathologic staging, the specialists go into the patient and examine the cancer. Pathologic staging is much more accurate and comprehensive; indeed, a substantial number of cancers originally assigned a low clinical stage are upgraded to higher pathological stages once the actual tumor is studied on a laboratory bench.

Dave will now have his cancer staged, and when the process is complete, his cancer will be given a tumor/node/metastasis (TNM) stage. The table and accompanying description indicate both clinical and pathological staging. It is understood that some categories in the table, such as the status of lymph nodes, are nearly impossible to determine in clinical staging. The category is included in the following description because node status is important in pathological staging.

Schematic diagram of primary tumor (T stage)

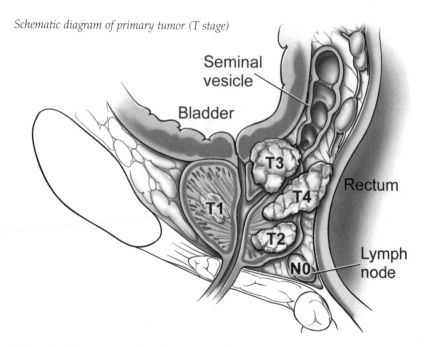

Schematic diagram of lymph node metastasis (N stage)

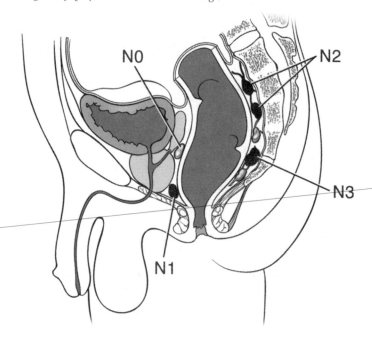

The Tumor-Nodes-Metastasis (TNM) system is used to estimate a tumor's extent. It helps practitioners predict the chance for cure, select appropriate treatment, and compare outcomes of different treatments.

THE TNM SYSTEM

Although medical technology has created some amazing tests and imaging devices, the body still holds secrets. Specialists attempt to gather as much information as they can because they want to make accurate treatment decisions. However, some information will always remain ambiguous despite the best efforts of specialist and machine.

Let's look more closely at the following tables. Stage T1a and T1b tumors are usually found while a man is undergoing surgery for

T – PRIMARY TUMOR STATUS	
Tx	Tumor cannot be assessed
T0	No evidence of a primary tumor
T1	Tumor not detectible by touch or imaging procedures
T1a	Incidental finding during other surgery; present in 5% of tissue or less
T1b	Incidental finding during other surgery; present in 5% of tissue or more
T1c	Found by needle biopsy because of a suspicious PSA
T2	Tumor confined within prostate
T2a	Involves half a lobe or less of prostate
T2b	Involves half a lobe
T2c	Involves both lobes
T3	Tumor extends through prostate capsule
T3a	Extends through one lobe
T3b	Extends through both lobes
T3c	Extends into seminal vesicles
T4	Tumor involves structures other than seminal vesicles
T4a	Invades bladder neck, external sphincter, or rectum
T4b	Invades muscles and/or pelvic wall

N – LYMPH NODE STATUS

NX	Nodes cannot be assessed
N0	No regional node metastasis
N1	Single node metastasis, 2 centimeters (cm) or less at largest point
N2	Single node metastasis, 2 cm to 5 cm at largest point, or multiple nodes, no larger than 5 cm at largest point
N3	Metastasis larger than 5 cm in any node

M – METASTATIC STATUS

MX	Metastasis cannot be assessed
M0	No distant metastasis
M1	Distant metastasis
M1a	Distant lymph node(s) involved
M1b	Bone(s) involved
M1c	Other site(s) involved

benign prostatic hyperplasia (BPH). It was noted earlier that prostates start growing again in middle age. When they reach the point that they are making urination problematic, one of the solutions is surgery. Sometimes this surgery turns up cancer. Surgeons who remove prostate tissue are not always able to recognize with the naked eye that the tissue is cancerous. So they send the tissue to the pathology lab for analysis, where a pathologist can spot cancerous cells under the microscope.

Another safeguard is that most men will have a PSA prior to undergoing surgery for BPH, and the presence of cancer will be assessed by a prostate ultrasound and needle biopsy prior to surgery in those whose PSA is considered worrisome. Furthermore, most techniques currently used for treating prostate enlargement do not involve any tissue removal.

In the PSA era, most newly diagnosed prostate cancer is Stage T1c.

Stage T2 describes tumors that may or may not involve a significant portion of the prostate, but are nonetheless confined to the prostate. Along with stage T1 cancers, these are the most curable tumors.

Stage T3 tumors have grown through the prostate capsule (a discontinuous layer on the outside of the prostate, similar to the rind on a citrus fruit, although much thinner) and may extend into the seminal vesicles, the glands adjacent to the prostate that produce most of the fluid that bathes and activates sperm. They can be cured, but they usually require more aggressive therapy than stage T1 and T2 tumors.

Stage T4 tumors are big. They have grown from the prostate to invade adjacent structures such as the bladder neck, rectum, and pelvic muscles. In the era of PSA screening, such tumors are rare.

Lymph node status and the presence or absence of metastatic disease can be difficult to obtain for clinical staging. Additional tests may or may not be employed, depending on the PSA, grade, and stage of the cancer.

Dave's initial staging assessment is T1cN0M0, which means that the tumor cannot be felt on DRE and has been detected only because of an elevated PSA. Thankfully, there is no evidence now that lymph nodes are involved or that the cancer has traveled beyond the prostate.

ADDITIONAL STAGING TECHNOLOGY

At this point, most doctors would sit down with Dave and discuss treatment options. In addition, the physician may seek more information about his cancer with additional imaging tests. Among these are computed tomography (CT) scans, endorectal coil magnetic resonance imaging (MRI), transrectal ultrasonography (TRUS), radionuclide bone scans, and ProstaScint imaging.

Computed Tomography Scans

Dave has a Gleason sum of 7 and has been clinically staged as having T1cN0M0 prostate cancer. His physician is recommending a computed tomography (CT) scan. Dave's Gleason sum put him just over the line into the category of men at risk for lymph node metastasis – the spreading of the cancer to the lymph nodes. The emphasis here is on the term "at risk." It doesn't mean that he has metastatic cancer. It means that his chances of developing metastatic disease are greater than those of men with a lower Gleason sum. This is one of the factors that will be considered when Dave and his doctor decide upon a course of therapy.

The CT scan Dave underwent showed his prostate to be slightly enlarged but not unusually so, at least not for men his age. It also appears that the lymph nodes are not enlarged. Although this is a good sign, it does not absolutely exclude the possibility that the lymph nodes contain some microscopic cancer.

Magnetic Resonance Imaging

This technology appears to be particularly useful in determining whether the tumor extends beyond the prostate capsule or whether it has invaded the seminal vesicles. The technology relies on disturbing the spin of hydrogen atoms in water, so tissues that contain significant amounts of water, such as growing tumors, become visible on MRI images. MRI also can be useful in determining whether the tumor is affecting the neurovascular bundles, an important issue for men considering radical prostatectomy. (This procedure is described in Chapter 6.)

MRI images can be obtained by either scanning the whole body or using an endorectal coil during the scan. In either instance, the patient lies on a table, which then moves through the MRI machine. An endorectal coil is a wire coil in a flexible plastic tube that is inserted into the rectum. The rectal coil helps focus the image on the prostate gland.

Radionuclide Bone Scans

Bone scans are used to determine whether the cancer has metasta-sized to the bone. PSA values greater than 10 ng/mL and high Gleason scores (8 to 10) show that a patient is at risk for metastasis.

The procedure begins with the intravenous administration of a radioisotope (a radioactive compound). The harmless compound releases signals that a sensitive detector identifies and collates into an image. The isotope used in bone scans tends to accumulate where bone cells are regenerating. All bone cells regenerate, but do so at a modest pace. But this pace vastly speeds up when the cells are troubled by a disease such as cancer. The accumulation of the isotope in areas of more intense regeneration will show up as hot spots on images.

Bone scans can provide invaluable information, but as with all the previously described diagnostic procedures, they are not perfect. Microscopic deposits of cancerous cells may lurk in the bones and fail to show up on the scan. Arthritis, recent and dated bone fractures, and certain infections can also speed up bone regeneration and show up as "hot spots" on the images.

ProstaScint Scan

ProstaScint, the name of a product made by the Cytogen Corporation, uses a radioactively labeled monoclonal antibody imaged by a technique known as "single-photon emission computed tomography," which combines advances in biology with advances in physics and displays the result on a CT machine.

The procedure uses a monoclonal antibody and indium 111, a radioactive isotope of a silvery metal similar to aluminum. The antibody is a unique protein that seeks out prostate cells and binds itself to another protein called "prostate specific membrane anti-gen" (PSMA), which is found almost exclusively on the surface of prostate cells. The slightly radioactive indium emits signals that are picked up by sensors to be funneled into a computer that creates an image.

CRUNCH TIME

Everything that can be clinically known about Dave's prostate and its cancer is now in his medical record (whether electronic, paper, or film). Information in his folder shows Dave's PSA is 5.8 ng/mL. The pathologist has graded the biopsied tissue from the cancer at a Gleason of 3 + 4 and the clinical stage is listed as T1cN0M0.

The doctor's receptionist calls Dave to set up an appointment and suggests that Dave's wife attend. It's time to talk about treatments.

THE SCIENCE BEHIND COMPUTED TOMOGRAPHY

The principles that underlie computed tomography (CT), sometimes called computer-assisted tomography (CAT), are relatively simple.

Near the end of the 19th century, a German scientist named Wilhelm Conrad Roentgen was exploring the strange properties of certain frequencies of light emitted by cathode-ray tubes. In 1895, he published a formal report on the rays and, because he was not too certain what they were, named them after the standard mathematical symbol for an unknown quantity – X. He received a Nobel Prize for his research.

X-rays are high-energy light waves. We can't see them, but they can penetrate living tissue. In some tissues, the x-rays produce a dark spot on an x-ray film. Denser tissues (such as bone) are more difficult to penetrate; they leave blank spaces on the film that appear white. For example, chest x-rays do not capture the ribcage, because the x-ray machine does not take a picture of the ribs. Instead, it takes a picture of everything but the ribs. That's why the bones appear white.

The next step is to get as much information from the x-rays as possible. This is done by focusing the x-rays, because narrow beams cast much sharper shadows. Narrowing the x-ray beam also sharpens the image. Encasing the x-ray in a massive donut allows it to rotate around a body and snap a tiny picture from a different angle every millisecond or so. As the emitter circles the body, the donut slides forward so that every circle covers a different portion of the anatomy. Receptors placed on the other side of the donut directly opposite the x-ray emitter capture the emerging x-ray and the information it carries and sends it to a computer, which organizes all the information into what is called a slice. In fact, tomography is a combination of the Greek words *tomos* (to slice or section) and *graphein* (to write).

MORE ON MRI

The original term for this medical technology is "nuclear magnetic resonance imaging," but the name was changed to avoid any negative connotations from the word "nuclear" and to prevent patients from associating the examination with radiation exposure.

One advantage of MRI over x-rays is that, according to current medical knowledge, MRI scans are harmless to patients. MRI uses strong magnetic fields and nonionizing radiation in the radio-frequency range. (CT scans and traditional x-rays involve doses of ionizing radiation).

Instead of ionizing radiation, radio-frequency waves are directed at protons (the nuclei of hydrogen atoms) in a strong magnetic field. The protons are first "agitated" and then "relaxed"; this action emits radio signals that are captured to form a computer-processed image. In the body, protons are most abundant in the hydrogen atoms of water (and tissues predominantly contain water) so that an MRI shows differences in water content and distribution in various body tissues. Even different types of tissue within the same organ, such as the gray and white matter of the brain, can easily be distinguished by this method.

Typically an MRI examination consists of two to six imaging sequences, each lasting up to 15 minutes. Each sequence shows a cross-section of the body in one of several planes (left to right, back to front, etc.). ◆

Chapter 5

Treating the Cancer

In the 1950s, about the time Dave was getting his first baseball glove, the primary therapy for prostate cancer was radical prostatectomy – taking out the cancer, the prostate, and the adjacent lymph nodes. The procedure worked then and still works today. Radical prostatectomy continues to be the gold standard by which all other procedures are judged for long-term efficacy. But since then, a number of radiation treatments have been introduced, along with a range of new surgical technologies and new approaches to old surgical procedures.

The challenge confronting Dave, his wife, and his doctor is to decide which procedure is best suited to Dave's clinical situation. Which method of treatment will produce the best long-term results with the most acceptable side effects for Dave?

Some procedures are not applicable to Dave's condition, but are viable choices for others. Let's examine the three primary treatment options currently available to men diagnosed with prostate cancer: active surveillance, surgery, and radiation therapy.

ACTIVE SURVEILLANCE

The original concept was termed "watchful waiting," but there is no waiting involved here. Today, we refer to it as "active surveillance," "expectant therapy," or "deferred therapy," because these phrases more accurately describe a proactive approach taken by men who may have low-grade cancer and older patients whose lives are more than likely to end for reasons other than prostate cancer.

It was noted earlier that most forms of prostate cancer are slow-growing and may take 10 to 15 years or longer before they begin to produce symptoms that would affect a man's quality of life. But for a man in his 70s or 80s, prostate surgery and other aggressive treatments are likely to be difficult, particularly if he is already beset with other health problems. For a man in his 80s, watching the cancer closely and following a pattern of routine checkups to monitor its progress may be the best idea.

Yet active surveillance is not the exclusive province of older men. Younger men with low-grade cancer also have this option, but it is not without certain risks. In 2005, a consortium of Scandinavian institutions reported on a study of 695 men who were diagnosed in 1989 with early prostate cancer. Their mean age was about 65. They were assigned by a flip of a coin ("randomized") to be watched or to undergo radical prostatectomy, so that 347 of them had surgery and 348 experienced "watchful waiting." After 10 years, the men who underwent surgery had substantial reductions in cancer progression, including lower risks of:

- Urinary and other symptoms resulting from tumor growth in the prostate
- Development of metastasis
- Need for other treatments such as hormones or radiation
- Death from prostate cancer

Furthermore (and somewhat unexpectedly) the study found that in terms of quality-of-life issues, there was no difference between the men who had surgery and those being managed by watchful waiting. The men who had surgery had problems with urinary control and potency; the watchful-waiting group had more urinary symptoms resulting from local tumor growth and worried about the possibility of dying of cancer. While the results were intriguing, the great majority of men in the study had cancers that were large enough to be felt upon digital rectal examination (DRE) but were not detected by PSA. This is important because today most newly diagnosed cancers are found only by PSA elevations and are less aggressive than those in the Scandinavian study. Thus, there is some uncertainty regarding whether the results of the study apply to most men diagnosed today.

Several published studies have examined active surveillance as a management strategy in men with PSA-detected cancers. In one study from the University of Toronto, at eight years after study entry, only 2 of 299 patients who chose active surveillance had died of prostate cancer and about two-thirds avoided any treatment at all. In a study of 38 men with very small-volume Gleason 6 tumors at Johns Hopkins, delaying surgery by two years did not affect the chance for cure as assessed by pathological assessment of the removed prostate compared to the circumstances of similar men who had surgery immediately after being diagnosed. While these early results are encouraging, it is still not clear who are the best candidates for surveillance because we cannot always tell whether even a low-grade cancer is going to "tread water" or progress, how long it is safe to wait without intervening, or whether delaying therapy will jeopardize the chance for cure in some or most patients. Furthermore, no studies have quantified the psychological toll that comes with knowing that you are living with an untreated cancer whose behavior is not fully predictable. These uncertainties highlight the need for developing better biologically based markers of cancer behavior that would allow doctors to distinguish between those tumors that need treatment and those that can be safely watched.

The American Cancer Society estimated that 234,460 new cases of prostate cancer would be diagnosed in the United States in 2006. Therefore, it would be a great help to a patient if, during his diagnosis, all the factors surrounding his disease could be punched into a computer that would spit out a recommended course of action.

Fortunately, there are some newly developed tools that can help guide a decision. Dr. Michael Kattan, chairman of the Cleveland Clinic Department of Quantitative Health Sciences, developed charts known as nomograms to predict the likelihood that a patient's tumor would have low biological aggressiveness (and not require immediate radical therapy).

Nomograms combine information from a patient's serum PSA, clinical stage, and Gleason grade to predict the probability that a man with prostate cancer has a nonaggressive tumor and does not need an operation.

Nomograms have a good discriminatory ability and may benefit the patient and clinician when various treatment options for prostate cancer are being considered. However, the American Cancer society stresses the importance of continued monitoring of the prostate, even if a nomogram concludes that little risk is involved – after all, things change.

Basically, a nomogram works like this: Using a combination of data from several studies that tracked the progression of prostate cancer in patients along with facts about the patient himself – his clinical tests, age, lifestyle choices, environmental influences, etc. – Kattan created a chart that was able to predict pretty accurately *before aggressive treatment began* what a patient might encounter in various situations, such as the likelihood of finding cancer with a biopsy or of finding indolent or organ-confined disease, the likelihood of cure after various treatments, and how the patient would respond to salvage radiotherapy.

The Kattan "Pre-operative" Nomogram

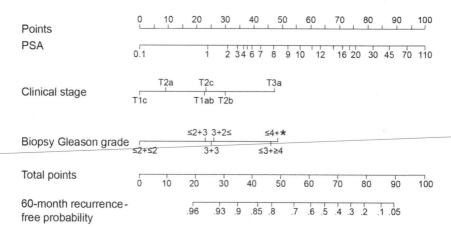

The nomogram calculates the likelihood of cure five years after radical prostatectomy, using the three most important factors available at diagnosis. For example, a man with a PSA of 6.5, a clinical stage T1c cancer, and Gleason 6 tumor totals 65 points and has an approximate 90 percent chance of being cancer-free five years after surgery.

Later, Kattan and others refined his predictive methodology by developing a postoperative nomogram that allows more accurate prediction of probability for prostate cancer recurrence for patients who had received radical prostatectomy, compared with the preoperative nomogram that many physicians had been using. The group studied 996 men with clinical stage T1a-T3c NXM0 prostate cancer who had been treated with radical prostatectomy and examined variables including pretreatment serum prostate specific antigen level, specimen Gleason sum, prostatic capsular invasion, surgical margin status, seminal vesicle invasion, and lymph node status. Physicians noted treatment failure resulting from clinical evidence of disease recurrence, a rising serum prostate specific antigen level (two measurements of 0.4 ng/mL or greater and rising), or initiation of adjuvant therapy, and found that the nomogram predictions appeared to be accurate. The study enabled physicians to develop a postoperative nomogram that can be used to predict the seven-year probability of disease recurrence among men treated with radical prostatectomy. (An even newer nomogram can predict the 10-year probability.)

SURGERY OR RADIATION?

Ask most surgeons for advice as to the best treatment for low-to-intermediate stage prostate cancer and they will without hesitation say surgery. Ask most radiation oncologists for advice as to the best treatment for low-to-intermediate stage prostate cancer and they will without hesitation say radiation treatments. The problem facing men like Dave is that in most instances, both groups of doctors are right.

Because there has yet to be a large definitive study that adequately compares prostatectomy to radiation therapy, making a head-to-head comparison of the two approaches is difficult. In addition, radical prostatectomy is usually recommended to younger men, while radiation therapy is recommended to older men who frequently have other health problems. In light of the age differences, it can be difficult to compare results, especially when those results may not be known for years. To further complicate the issue, results of both procedures are often spread over large numbers of men. They will tell Dave *the probability* of how well one procedure or another works in all men between the ages of 52 and 65, but they will not tell *exactly* how well each procedure might work specifically for him.

This makes the consultation between Dave and his doctor very important. Outcome predictions can be made that are tailored to Dave and the "clinical" characteristics of his cancer, which are those aspects of the cancer that can be determined without a thorough surgical examination. But once the surgeon sees the cancer up close, he and the pathologist who will study the organ later may come up with a different set of "pathologic" characteristics. Because, after all, outcomes predicted by pathologic characteristics are substantially more accurate than those predicted by clinical characteristics.

The approach Dave should take in making a therapeutic decision is to learn as much as he can about the advantages and disadvantages of each procedure and choose the one he feels best suits his desires and situation. How does Dave do this? By asking his doctor lots of questions and by using a nomogram, which could help predict the likelihood of a cure.

RADICAL PROSTATECTOMY

Radical prostatectomy is a well-established and safe procedure, and intra-operative and post-operative complications are rare.

Radical prostatectomy involves removing the entire prostate, seminal vesicles, and adjacent lymph nodes (if necessary). The prostate can be reached from two approaches. In a retropubic prostatectomy, the initial incision is made in the lower abdomen. In a perineal prostatectomy, the initial incision is made in the perineum, the bridge of flesh between the scrotum and anus.

Regardless of the approach, the procedure typically lasts from 90 minutes up to three hours and may be conducted under general, spinal, or epidural anesthesia. Both open procedures – retropubic and perineal – may require hospital stays of up to two days. While the connection between the bladder and urethra heals, a catheter (thin, flexible tube) is placed into the penis to drain the urine for one to two weeks.

There is a subset of prostatectomies categorized as "minimally invasive" procedures. Laparoscopic and robot-assisted prostatectomy, which involve less blood loss, entail placing several tubes through incisions about 8 to 10 mm long (a pencil is 8 mm thick).

In robot-assisted prostatectomies, the instruments are moved by a robot controlled by the surgeon. The movement at the working end of the instruments accurately mimics the movements of the surgeon's hands; if the surgeon moves his hand to the right, the scalpel moves right. Robotic surgery also offers movement reduction – a surgeon may move a hand three inches to the right, but the scalpel may move only one inch: a 3:1 movement reduction. This allows for accurate and fine movement of instruments when necessary. One advantage of robotic surgery is that the surgeon can use a monitor to get a real-life 3D view of the operative field, as opposed to a flat 2D perspective offered to the laparoscopic surgeon.

The best way to choose how to have the prostate removed is by investigating the experience of the surgeon. Learn the results he or she has achieved for similar patients. The most important outcomes after prostatectomy are the rate of positive margins, the rapidity and completeness of return of urinary control, and the return of potency. These outcomes are dependent upon the skill and experience of the surgeon, not which technique is used to remove the prostate. A recent study has shown that for the same grade and stage of disease, if the surgery is performed by a surgeon who has carried out more than 1,000 procedures, likelihood of cure after radical prostatectomy is 10 percent higher than after surgery carried out by a surgeon who has performed 250, and 30 percent higher than after surgery done by someone who has performed fewer than 50.

Nerve-sparing prostatectomies can be conducted as open or laparoscopic procedures. Up until the 1980s, the prostate was removed with little concern for the nerves that run along each side of the prostate to the penis, where they receive the stimuli that promotes and holds erections through ejaculation and climax. When the nerves were severed, impotence followed. This occurred primarily because the precise location of the nerves was not known then. But even if the location of the nerves had been known, in that era most men had large cancers that would have required removal of the nerves anyway in order to get all the cancer out.

All that changed in the early 1980s with the development of nerve-sparing prostatectomies by Patrick Walsh of Johns Hopkins Hospital. What was then considered a remarkable procedure is now common for men like Dave, whose disease is confined within the prostate capsule. Again, the results of the procedure vary among surgeons. Today, for most men who have early-stage tumors detected by PSA, the good news is that in experienced hands, the nerve bundles can be saved in almost 100 percent of cases. Even though the nerve bundles can be safely dissected away from the prostate, they do get bruised from handling during surgery. Such nerve tissue is slow to heal and in most men, potency does not usually return immediately and may take up to 24 months to recover. Fortunately, drugs that enhance potency, such as sildenifil and the other PDE5 inhibitors, can expand the opportunity for full recovery. Drugs that helped the nerves heal faster when tested in animal models are now being studied in humans.

Incontinence is another complication associated with prostatectomy. Most men will experience some degree of incontinence in the days immediately following removal of the catheter, which generally heals in six to 12 weeks. Less than 10 percent of patients will require long-term use of a pad for stress incontinence (a spurt of a drop or two of urine that occurs when coughing, sneezing, swinging a golf club, and similar activities result in abdominal straining). In the rare instance when persistent leakage is a problem, one of several minor surgical procedures can be performed to correct it.

RADIATION THERAPY

Dave is eligible for radiation therapy. This therapy is indicated for men with organ-confined low-stage disease, as well as more locally advanced (stage T3 or some stage T4) tumors.

Radiation treatments exploit one of the few weaknesses of cancer cells. These cells multiply at a much higher rate than normal cells, and it is during this replication process that their dividing DNA is sensitive to destruction by radiation. This particular weakness allows radiation oncologists to tailor radiation dosages to levels that will destroy cancer cells, but leave most normal cells unharmed.

There are two primary radiation therapies for prostate cancer: external beam radiation therapy and brachytherapy. External beam radiation treatment is noninvasive. In brachytherapy, a minimally invasive procedure, a needle is used to implant tiny radioactive seeds in tumors.

EXTERNAL BEAM RADIATION TREATMENT

As the name implies, a tightly controlled beam of radiation is focused on the tumor. Radiation treatments are painless; the experience has been likened to getting an x-ray.

External beam technologies can be subdivided into categories based on the energy source used to generate the beam (electrons or protons) and the computer-assisted planning technology used to aim the beam at the prostate. Electron beams use gamma radiation to destroy cells, whereas proton beam radiation uses a tightly focused beam of protons. Proton generators, otherwise known as cyclotrons, are large, relatively new, and expensive devices. Not all hospitals or medical institutions may have proton beam technology.

Both radiation-beam technologies rely on computers to acquire images of tumors, design delivery patterns, and control the beams as the radiation is delivered. The computers analyze the information they are given from CT scans and other imaging technologies, and present oncologists with one or more suggested treatment plans.

The oncologist spreads the radiation treatments over a number of weeks, fine-tuning the treatment plan as newer information about the tumor becomes known. The tumor cells perish slowly over the following several months.

The current state of the art for radiation delivery is one of several "conformal" techniques that shape the radiation beam in three dimensions to conform to the shape of the prostate. This allows very high doses to be delivered to the prostate and improves the chances for cure while minimizing the scatter to surrounding normal tissues (primarily the rectum and bladder), thus minimizing side effects. Intensity-modulated radiation therapy, which delivers precise radiation doses, is the most recent innovation in conformal therapies.

SIDE EFFECTS

Despite all precautions, a certain amount of radiation is going to strike healthy tissues and organs around the prostate. Because of this, some patients may experience bowel toxicity – tenderness in the rectum and diarrhea. Other side effects include:

- Bladder irritation that appears as a sense of urgency to urinate or urination that is frequent or painful
- Proctitis or irritable bowel
- Erectile and ejaculatory dysfunction

Sildenifil and similar compounds have shown significant benefit in restoring erectile function impaired by radiation treatments.

COMBINED RADIATION AND HORMONE THERAPY

The prostate is a male gland nourished by male hormones (androgens), principally testosterone. Approximately 85 percent of all testosterone is produced in the testes, with most of the remaining 15 percent produced in the adrenal glands that rest atop the kidneys.

Dr. Charles Huggins demonstrated in 1941 that depriving the glands of testosterone causes the prostate to shrink. Huggins later won a Nobel Prize for his work showing that testosterone deprivation caused regression of metastatic tumors.

The prostate can be deprived of testosterone through castration or with compounds that either block the hormone production or interfere with the hormone's activity. Hormone therapy can be a primary treatment for advanced and metastatic prostate cancer, and a secondary treatment for organ-confined prostate cancer.

Hormone therapy is known as neoadjuvant therapy when it is used *before* a definitive treatment and as adjuvant therapy when used to supplement or to *follow* a definitive treatment. The idea behind using hormone therapy as a neoadjuvant treatment is that depriving the malignant cells of the compounds needed for growth before they are treated with radiation makes them more susceptible to radiation. Similarly, depriving these cells of growth factors after they have been weakened by radiation may speed their death. The combined treatment is often chosen when the cancer is known to have spread beyond the prostate but remains contained in adjacent structures and tissues. Hormone therapy can be used with either external beam radiation treatment or brachytherapy; several studies have shown that for high-grade or high-stage tumors, hormone therapy plus external beam radiation results in higher cure rates than external beam radiation alone.

BRACHYTHERAPY

Brachytherapy delivers radiation to a tumor from the inside out, thereby minimizing the radiation tissues and organs outside the prostate. As with an external beam, it is usually recommended for men with organ-confined tumors.

In 1999, up to a third of men with localized prostate cancer opted for brachytherapy, a one-time treatment that usually is completed on an outpatient basis. With this procedure, the prostate is carefully imaged by means of transrectal ultrasound. Once the size and shape of the prostate are determined, tiny radioactive seeds are placed at specific locations inside the prostate. Each seed is surrounded with a radiation aura that is deadly to cancerous cells. (Picture the seeds in a grape; each aura would be shaped like a grape, but smaller). The trick to designing an effective brachytherapy is to insert the seeds into the prostate so that the shapes of their auras match the shape of the prostate. Computers are used to generate a "plan" that includes the number and location of the needles and seeds for optimum dosing. The needles that deliver the seeds are guided into the prostate using ultrasound technology. The commonest form of brachytherapy is low-dose rate (LDR) using permanently implanted iodine (125I) or palladium (103Pd) seeds.

> Once the size and shape of the prostate are determined, tiny radioactive seeds are placed at specific locations inside the prostate.

High dose rate (HDR) brachytherapy is another brachytherapy method. Under this procedure, a high dose rate source (often iridium 192) is delivered to the tumor. The advantage of this treatment is that it shortens radiation exposure because all the radiation is expended within 48 hours.

There is no evidence that one form of brachytherapy is better than another with respect to cure rates, and as is the case for radical prostatectomy, the degree of experience of the team performing the procedure may be the most important factor to consider in the choice of how to treat the tumor.

The side effects associated with brachytherapy include swelling and/or inflammation of the prostate in the days immediately following insertion of the seeds, typically resulting in irritative voiding symptoms. Occasionally, persistent urinary retention, rectal urgency, bowel movement frequency, rectal bleeding or ulceration, and prostatorectal fistulas – holes between the prostate and the rectum – may occur. These symptoms affect less than 10 percent of the men being treated, and serious symptoms such as fistulas occur in less than 1 percent.

HOW DO I KNOW WHETHER IT WORKED?

No therapy comes with a guarantee. Every man treated for prostate cancer will be monitored for the possibility of cancer recurrence for the rest of his life.

Patients who pursue a course of active surveillance will have their PSA monitored at regular checkups, which will include blood tests to monitor serum creatinine, digital rectal examinations (DREs), and ultrasound. As noted earlier, PSA is a somewhat fickle compound that may give over- or under-inflated readings. Isolated elevations of the antigen may or may not spell trouble, but a consistently rising PSA may indicate a need for intervention.

A radical prostatectomy is designed to remove all possible tissue that would be susceptible to malignant change. PSA should disappear completely from a man's system after surgery if all the cancer was removed. Any PSA that appears is being produced by prostate tissue missed by the treatment, and there is a strong likelihood that the tissue is malignant. This phenomenon is known as biochemical relapse.

One problem with using PSA to monitor the success of a therapy is the exquisite sensitivity of current tests. Ultrasensitive PSA assays can detect the antigen down to levels as low as 0.0098 ng/mL. The general rule of thumb is that a PSA reading of 0.2 ng/mL and rising constitutes biochemical relapse. The speed at which the PSA is rising (velocity) and/or its "doubling time" (the time it takes to go from 0.2 to 0.4 to 0.8, for example) can help determine whether the cancer has recurred locally or has become metastatic, so appropriate treatments can be started. Doctors are learning more about the prognostic value of PSA recurrence from large-scale studies suggesting that men whose PSA doubles rapidly (less than every three months) are at high risk of developing metastasis and dying and need additional therapy, while those with long doubling times (more than 12 months) are at low risk and may be safely observed.

After brachytherapy or radiation treatments, PSA will begin to fall during the next few weeks to months until it hits its lowest point, called the nadir. However, PSA may not fall all the way to <0.2 as it does after surgery, since remaining normal prostate tissue unaffected by the radiation still makes some PSA. What constitutes PSA failure after brachytherapy or external radiation therapy is therefore controversial; a recent consensus has suggested that a definition of PSA nadir + 2 (i.e., a PSA that has risen to a total of 2 ng/ml after reaching its lowest, or nadir, point) is the best predictor of whether local or distant recurrences will develop.

There is general agreement on two issues about PSA after radiation-based approaches. First, studies have shown that the longer it takes for PSA to reach its lowest level, the better the prognosis. Second, up to one-third of patients after brachytherapy have a rise and fall in PSA that is not indicative of cancer recurrence – this "PSA bounce" typically occurs in younger patients 18 to 24 months after therapy and resolves itself spontaneously and without any further treatment.

OTHER THERAPIES

Cryosurgery (or cryotherapy) is not a common procedure, but it is available at a number of institutions. It involves placing a probe into the prostate. The temperature at the tip of the probe plummets, causing adjacent prostate tissue to freeze and perish. The therapy was more prevalent in the past, but difficulty controlling the extent of freezing (the so-called iceball formation), which resulted in tissue destruction, caused it to fall from favor. The therapy is enjoying a resurgence, owing to improved control of the freezing process and improvements in imaging technologies that allow the amount of tissue being destroyed by the iceball to be closely observed. It is typical for the tumor to be frozen, allowed to thaw, and frozen again.

Cryosurgery offers certain advantages. It is minimally invasive and may be repeated if there is residual malignant tissue or the tumor begins to grow again. Cryosurgery also can be used as a "salvage" therapy to destroy residual cancer following prostatectomy or radiation therapy. Studies of cryotherapy using newer techniques and technologies are rather young. As noted earlier, it takes years for the effectiveness of a prostate cancer therapy to be evaluated with confidence.

The side effects of cryotherapy include urinary incontinence, impotence, and prostatitis (inflammation of the prostate). About half the men who undergo the procedure experience one of these problems. As noted, advancing technology has given the procedure a new life, and research is continuing to add improvements and refinements that may boost the efficacy of the procedure and reduce the incidence of side effects. ◆

Chapter 6

When the Cancer
Fights Back

Although prostate cancer is among the most treatable of all malignancies, even the best therapies can fail. There is no way of knowing who will suffer recurrence. Though it is true that men with more aggressive disease (those with higher Gleason scores, higher PSA levels, and tumor growth) are at greater risk for failure, it is just as true that many aggressive tumors can be cured.

And, although rare, even a low-risk tumor can occasionally return.

What are the chances of that happening? One study reported that 95 percent of the men who completed radiation therapy and received a post-treatment PSA of less than 0.5 were cancer-free at five years, and 84 percent were cancer-free at 10 years. A 2006 study of approximately 5,000 men across the country found that patients treated with a higher dose of radiation had a better chance of achieving a lower PSA score and were less likely to see their prostate cancer return. In fact, patients with the lowest PSA scores experienced an eight-year disease-free survival rate of 75 percent, compared with only 18 percent for those with the highest PSA scores. Patients who had the lower PSA scores also had a 97 percent metastasis-free survival rate versus 73 percent for those with the highest PSA scores.

Detecting a PSA rising does not necessarily mean that the prostate cancer has returned and spread (metastasized) to other areas of the body. In fact, in the first 10 years after surgery, the fortunes of men with a detectable PSA are little different from those who remain PSA-free. We took a close look at this at Cleveland Clinic and found that the 10-year survival rates for patients with detectable PSA was 88 percent, compared to 93 percent for those without detectable PSA. Moreover, 74 percent of the men who did show detectable PSA were metastasis-free at 10 years. This heartening finding allowed us to conclude that at 10 years, following a radical prostatectomy for localized disease, patients with PSA recurrence have an excellent overall survival rate equal to that of men with no detectable PSA. Furthermore, recent Cleveland Clinic data showed that at 10 years after surgery or external beam radiation, patients had only a 2 percent chance of dying of prostate cancer.

In a 2002 study, Dr. Anthony D'Amico, an associate professor of radiation oncology at Harvard Medical School, followed 381 people to see whether he could identify success factors in men who underwent external radiation therapy for prostate cancer. He divided the men into three groups: high, intermediate, and low risk of death from prostate cancer, based on pretreatment factors including T stage, PSA at diagnosis, and Gleason grade. The study found that PSA scores that doubled in one year or less was an almost sure predictor of death. Of the 18 men in his study who showed such a rise, 17 (95 percent) of them died because the cancer spread to their bones. The findings showed that those whose PSAs double in less than a year require quick, aggressive intervention.

Furthermore, of the 381 men in the study, almost half (45 percent) of those at high risk died of their prostate cancer within 10 years. About a quarter (27 percent) died from heart disease, stroke, complications of diabetes, or other causes. But keep this in mind: At the time of their diagnoses, the median age of these men was 73. The risk of dying of prostate cancer for men in the intermediate-risk group was 6 percent. And for those in the low-risk group, the risk was zero.

Still, metastatic cancer does appear. It is not new cancer, but a remnant of the old cancer: cells that drifted from the primary tumor in the prostate before it was removed or destroyed. This is why larger tumors and tumors that have expanded beyond the prostatic capsule have a higher risk of becoming metastatic. The more aggressive a tumor is, the greater its tendency to shed cells. These tumor cells move into the lymph nodes or bloodstream and are ferried throughout the body. Although these cells can lodge anywhere – lung, liver, brain – and begin to grow, the most common sites for prostate cancer metastasis are the lymph nodes and bones. It is estimated that more than 90 percent of all prostate cancer metastases occur in bones. This is prostate cancer, not bone cancer. The parent cell that seeded the cancer is a drifting malignant prostate cell that lodges in the bone, begins to multiply, and creates a metastasis.

DIAGNOSES

When rising PSA appears, doctors and specialists try to determine whether the recurrence is confined to the prostate area or has spread into the bones, the lymph nodes in and around the pelvis, and in soft tissue adjacent to the prostate.

Symptoms related to the cancer rarely appear before PSA begins to rise. As the tumor progresses, patients can experience bone pain or sciatica, and very rarely paralysis in the legs as a result of spinal cord compression, which is sometimes accompanied by lethargy and weight loss. But in the majority of instances, the spread of the disease will be signaled by rising PSA levels. This is an indication that more testing is needed to determine how much disease is present and where it might lie. Whatever those tests find will determine how the cancer will be fought a second time and which therapy might be best this time around.

Every disease has its own tests and examinations that are meant to describe every aspect of disease. The one for advanced prostate cancer includes a series of blood tests and imaging studies that serve two purposes – to show in general terms how much disease there is and where it might lie, and to serve as a benchmark that will let physicians monitor the effect that therapy is having on the disease. There is no one therapy for advanced prostate cancer, but rather a course or series of therapies that are used as the cancer changes.

LAB AND IMAGING STUDIES

Blood tests can provide a wealth of information about the character of the cancer and how well various organs are functioning. Also, a variety of markers can shed light on what is going on.

Imaging tests may include a bone scan, a chest x-ray, computed tomography (CT) or MRI of the abdomen and pelvis, and an imaging technique known as ProstaScint. The ProstaScint scan's value is that it sometimes can differentiate between local and distant recurrences. This is a very clever technical trick. The test involves injecting a radiolabeled monoclonal antibody – a small protein that will find and stick to only one particular antigen. Every cell line has its own characteristic set of antigens. In ProstaScint imaging, the antigen to which the antibody binds is prostate specific membrane antigen (PSMA). If all prostate tissue has been removed by prostatectomy or destroyed by radiation, there should be no PSMA for the antibody to bind to. When the antibody finds PSMA, it will bind to it in little clumps, and since a small bit of harmless radioactive tracer is attached to the antibody, the clumps will show up as dark spots on the film.

When PSA rises above 10 ng/mL or symptoms are present, scintigraphy, also known as a bone scan, might be called for to detect skeletal metastasis. The entire skeleton is surveyed for evidence of metastasis. Because most testing is initiated long before PSA reaches these levels, bone scans are seldom the first test employed.

Bone scintigraphy involves the intravenous injection of a radiolabeled tracer, which is detected on film or video. The tracer, Tc-99m MDP (technetium-99m methylene diphosphonate), binds to regions of high osteoblastic activity. Osteoblasts are cells that form bone tissue, and they kick into high gear when malignant prostate cells lodge in the bone. The problem is that there are other processes that encourage osteoblasts to kick it up a notch, including trauma from fractures, infection, and degenerative joint diseases such as arthritis. While scintigraphy is sensitive enough to pick up this activity, it is not so good at determining what exactly is causing the activity. This is why if bone scintigraphy picks up something, an additional test such as CT or magnetic resonance imaging is sometimes used to confirm the presence of bone disease.

Computed tomography of the abdomen and pelvic regions is sometimes used to identify local disease, but the technology is not that sensitive; it can often miss disease that is present. CT can detect enlarged lymph nodes and the occasional circumstance where the tumor spreads to visceral organs, but it cannot detect microscopic disease.

TREATING RECURRENT PROSTATE CANCER

Local recurrent disease can be treated by removing whatever tissue might be left (salvage prostatectomy), by freezing it (salvage cryotherapy), or by using radiation (salvage radiotherapy). The choice of treatment involves factors such as the initial treatment (prostatectomy or radiation) and the location of the disease.

Radiation therapy can be considered if the recurrent disease falls within an area that can be targeted with the radiation beam. Prostatectomy or cryosurgery may be considered for men who have undergone external beam radiation therapy or brachytherapy. Salvage prostatectomy is appropriate when the initial cancer is confined to the prostate and remains confined to the prostate. In general, these cases occur in men with a low to intermediate Gleason sum (equal to or less than 6), a pretreatment PSA of 10ng/mL or less, and a T1c to T2a tumor stage at the initial diagnosis.

METASTATIC PROSTATE CANCER

Since Dr. Charles Huggins' groundbreaking discovery that depriving the glands of testosterone causes the prostate to shrink, androgen deprivation therapy (ADT) – denying prostate cancer cells male hormones – has become an established therapy for metastatic cancer. ADT buys time, but it will not cure anyone. Eventually, the cancer will become independent of hormones. It will grow and spread whether or not testosterone is present.

Evidence suggests that for those with established metastasis, ADT may prolong life and reduce cancer-related complications, such as ureteral obstruction and bone fractures. ADT also causes side effects such as hot flashes, loss of libido, reduced muscle mass, mild anemia, and osteoporosis, all of which can have a substantial impact on a patient's quality of life. Recent evidence suggests that ADT can also cause metabolic syndrome and increase the risk of cardiovascular disease, so that its use in men with a detectable PSA and no evidence of metastasis should be carefully considered. To help identify those at risk of these side effects and prevent their occurrence, men starting on hormone therapy should have a battery of tests including EKG, lipid profile, fasting blood sugar, and bone density (DEXA) scan at the time they start hormone therapy. Treatable risk factors should be addressed by dietary and lifestyle changes, use of oral drugs such as statins, and calcium/vitamin D supplements or bisphosphonates.

Several studies investigating combined androgen blockade (CAB), which combines hormone therapy with either chemical castration or orchiectomy, and bicalutamide showed promising results for men with advanced prostate cancer. Prostate cancer growth is stimulated by male hormones, or androgens, most notably testosterone. The goal of hormone treatment is to prevent the stimulation of cancer cells by testosterone. Without testosterone, the tumor is, in a sense, starved so that it either stops growing, grows more slowly, or in some cases even shrinks. However, the testicles are not the body's only source of testosterone: The adrenal glands manufacture a substance that can be converted into testosterone.

Therefore, even when production by the testes is suppressed, prostate cancer can still be fed by small amounts of testosterone derived from the adrenal glands. Combined androgen blockade may prolong life by about three months in men with metastatic prostate cancer, but it produces significantly more side effects and worse quality of life than either medical or surgical castration alone produces.

Eventually, all metastatic cancer will become indifferent to the absence of testosterone and begin to grow again. This is inevitable.

This cancer is called androgen-independent cancer or hormone-refractory cancer. At this point, drugs such as mitoxantrone and docetaxel are used to induce regression of the cancer. Both of these drugs can result in significant palliation of bone pain and other symptoms of advanced cancer, and docetaxel has been shown to prolong life in men with bone metastasis that is resistant to ADT.

THE THERAPIES

ADT can be divided into traditional and nontraditional categories. Traditional ADT includes orchiectomy (castration), luteinizing hormone-releasing hormone agonists (hormones that discourage the production of testosterone), and a combination of both. Nontraditional therapies include intermittent androgen ablation, anti-androgen monotherapy, and anti-androgen therapy combined with 5-alpha-reductase inhibitors. A brief explanation of these terms follows.

Orchiectomy. Although orchiectomy is considered to be the "gold standard" method of androgen ablation in that it produces sudden and absolute reductions in testosterone, the psychological impact of castration and the procedure's irreversibility cause many to hesitate.

In this procedure, surgeons remove the testicles by making about a four-inch incision along the "bikini line" through the lower abdomen or through the scrotum. Once the incision has been made, the surgeon snips the spermatic cords and stitches the incision closed. The procedure takes about 30 to 45 minutes and may be performed on an outpatient basis or with an overnight hospital stay.

Luteinizing hormone-releasing hormone. Luteinizing hormone-releasing hormone (LHRH), which is produced in the hypothalamus, causes the pituitary gland to produce luteinizing hormone, which then stimulates testicular production of testosterone. Stop the LHRH and you stop the manufacture of testosterone.

This is accomplished by introducing LHRH agonists into the body. Agonists are compounds that look like the original compound but function more like decoys. LHRH agonists bind to molecular receptors in the pituitary gland, but do not prompt the cells to produce testosterone. Because the cellular receptors are plugged with the biological decoys, the real LHRH has no place to bind and becomes ineffectual.

There is an important difference between agonists and antagonists. The latter drugs simply block molecular receptors. LHRH agonists prevent production of testosterone in prostate cells, but they have no effect on testosterone production governed by the pituitary glands, which make luteinizing hormone (LH). Antagonists block the pituitary's production of LH and are also used to suppress what is called the "flare phenomenon," a surge of testosterone production, which may appear in up to 10 percent of men or more soon after LHRH agonist therapy is begun. The flare can have a number of bothersome effects. It can exacerbate bone pain and other bone-associated symptoms in patients with skeletal metastasis and can accelerate spinal cord compression in those with spinal disease.

Although clinically evident flare is uncommon, some physicians begin an oral antiandrogen 10 to 30 days before LHRH agonist treatment is started. The use of the antiandrogen blocks the effect of the testosterone surge caused by the LHRH *agonist* and prevents symptomatic flare. Long term use of an antiandrogen and LHRH agonist together is called "combined androgen blockade" (CAB) and is described in detail below.

Intermittent androgen ablation. Intermittent androgen ablation is thought to improve quality of life by reducing the side effects of ADT. In animal testing, the therapy appeared to prolong the time that metastatic cells are kept at bay by androgen deprivation. The therapy is administered in pulses or by a rhythm that spans months. The therapy begins with the administration of either LHRH agonists or antiandrogens. When PSA and testosterone levels fall to predetermined levels, the therapy is stopped. This usually takes about six months. PSA levels and testosterone are then closely monitored and when they rise again to a certain level, the androgen deprivation therapy is reinitiated.

There is a growing acceptance of this approach, but formal guidelines to recommend how the therapy should be administered have yet to be developed. The Committee on the Management of Disseminated Prostate Cancer recommended that the most appropriate patients for intermittent therapy were men 70 and older who wished to maintain sexual functioning and a higher quality of life, men under 70 with Gleason scores of 6 or lower, and men with local or biochemical recurrence after radiotherapy or radical prostatectomy.

Antiandrogens are used to prevent or moderate flare phenomenon, but they may also have a role in more comprehensive therapy. There are two categories of antiandrogens: steroidal and nonsteroidal. Cyproterone acetate and megestrol acetate are steroidal. The three nonsteroidal antiandrogens are bicalutamide, flutamide, and nilutamide. There have been a number of clinical trials with these agents, and the trials have produced different outcomes, so comparing one therapy to another is difficult. The Prostate Cancer Trials Collaborative Group looked at most of these trials and concluded that the addition of an antiandrogen to ADT by orchiectomy or LHRH agonists improved five-year survival by about 3 percent.

In common practice only the nonsteroidals are now used, and the market is dominated by Casodex (bicalutamide) because of side effects associated with the others drugs.

Antiandrogen monotherapy is an androgen-suppressing therapy that produces fewer sexual side effects than accompany CAB. Its use is generally restricted to those with a rising PSA and no detectable metastasis; antiandrogen monotherapy is not appropriate for those with demonstrable metastasis.

Bisphosphonates are drugs that strengthen bones and reduce high levels of calcium in the blood. They were initially developed to treat osteoporosis but have found a role in treating bone problems caused by prostate cancer and its varied therapies, particularly androgen deprivation. It is estimated that men on ADT may lose up to 5 percent of their bone mineral density after one year on the therapy. The cancer itself affects bones, and men with cancer in their bones suffer pain, fractures, and spinal compression. They frequently have to undergo surgery to repair these problems. Bisphosphonates provide pain relief and slow bone deterioration; they may even slow the progress of the cancer.

However, reports of significant side effects, especially osteonecrosis (loss of blood to bone tissue) of the jaw, have dulled enthusiasm for their use. Also, these medications are poorly absorbed and any food in the stomach will reduce the amount of drug that the body absorbs. Some bisphosphonates are given by IV infusion.

Radiation treatments may provide a palliative effect for those who seek pain relief. "Palliative" means that the pain and other symptoms are reduced, but the treatment has no effect on disease progression itself. Local radiation targets specific locations known to harbor metastases. Radiation also can be delivered by radioisotopes administered intravenously. These small molecules accumulate in tumors in bone and slow the progress of the disease.

> Radiation treatments may provide a palliative effect for those who seek pain relief.

Three radioisotopes are being used in this approach, and more are being studied. The available isotopes are phosphorus-32, strontium-89, and samarium-153. Each has unique properties, and one has not been proven better than the other. For instance, strontium-189 and phosphorus-32 achieve good penetration into the bone (between 2.4 and 2.7 mm). But strontium has a half-life of 50.5 days, and phosphorus has a half-life of 14.3 days. (Half-life is the amount of time it takes for an isotope to lose half its strength.) In strontium's case, this means that it is delivering a relatively powerful dose of radiation to cancer cells for more than seven weeks. This might be thought of as a good thing, but the isotope is also delivering the same amount of radiation to normal tissue during this period, which can result in depressed blood counts and limit the amount of chemotherapy that can be given (since the latter can also depress blood counts). Samarium-153, on the other hand, has a half-life of less than two days. It works quickly, but its penetration is reduced (about 0.55 mm).

The choice of an isotope is therefore dependent on the nature of the disease, preference and experience of the oncologist, and preference of the patient. Yet radioisotopes are rarely used because they suppress bone marrow function and limit the possible use of chemotherapy.

EVOLVING THERAPIES

Perhaps because prostate cancer is so common, many new therapies and therapeutic approaches are slowly making their way through the medical trial system. These therapies will be discussed briefly in Chapter 8, "Clinical Trials." ◆

Chapter 7

Preventing Prostate Cancer

Dave might have spared himself a lot of grief over his health had he practiced some simple preventive measures, such as exercising more often, paying more attention to his diet, and choosing foods that help prevent cancer.

Dave is like most of us. During his youth, he ate what his parents put on the table, and as he grew older began eating more processed and fast food. It was faster and easiser to take a meal out of the freezer and pop it into a microwave oven, or to open a can and heat its contents over a stove, than to prepare fresh produce from scratch. Unfortunately, those "easy-to-heat" foods often contain lots of sodium, fat, and chemical preservatives that, over time, just don't prove as good for you as fruits and vegetables, which are loaded with vitamins and other natural nutrients.

There appears to be little question now that some foods exert strong protective effects against prostate cancer and other cancers. But the challenge for researchers and investigators is to find out which foods are best and how much of each one is needed to produce the greatest benefit.

For instance, a few years ago a perfectly legitimate news article reported that pizza reduces the risk of prostate cancer. This was not a jest. The article, which reported on a study in a highly respected cancer journal, stated, "Analysis of the collected data clearly showed that men with a high consumption of tomato sauce, tomatoes, and pizza have a significantly lower risk of developing prostate cancer." This is the sort of thing that drives epidemiologists, who study the relationship of diseases to society and segments of society, crazy. Here are the first questions they would ask regarding such a study: What kind of pizza were the men eating? How much tomato sauce was on it? How much garlic (another cancer-fighting food) was on the pizza?

This illustrates the problems researchers have in figuring out what is good for a person and what puts a person at risk. That is, everything needs to be quantifiably proven. Studies have shown that both tomatoes and garlic may lower the risk of prostate cancer. Yet tomato juice, as tasty as it may be over ice, does not appear to offer protection. In order for tomatoes to exert a preventive influence, they must first be lightly cooked in oil – in other words, they must be turned into tomato sauce. Hence, the connection to pizza. One of the key nutrients in tomatoes is lycopene, but for it to be effectively absorbed by humans, it must first be sizzled in oil. That is what the researchers theorized.

> In order for tomatoes to exert a preventive influence, they must first be lightly cooked in oil – in other words, they must be turned into tomato sauce.

The point is that any natural food or herb contains thousands of compounds. The amounts of these compounds vary significantly from batch to batch and can vary even more when they are prepared for marketing. When a nutritionist, herbalist, or anyone else says that studies have shown that a certain fruit, vegetable, or herb cures this or prevents that, take the advice with a grain of salt. (In fact, watch your salt intake, too.) Diets that promote health and prevent disease do so only when they are followed with a certain degree of consistency. You cannot offset six days of fatty double cheeseburgers by eating a carrot on Sunday. Furthermore, it is not clear that dietary changes later in life will have any protective effect, and there are no conclusive data to suggest that dietary changes or nutritional supplements have any effect on a cancer once it has been diagnosed.

However, there are a number of substances – some created in a lab and some grown in a garden – that may lower the risk of prostate cancer. Among these are finasteride, selenium, vitamin E, vitamin D, soy, lycopene, green tea, COX-2 inhibitors, and red wine.

FINASTERIDE

Finasteride is a type-2 5-alpha-reductase inhibitor initially developed to reduce prostate size in men with benign prostatic hyperplasia. Five-alpha reductase is an enzyme that converts testosterone into its more potent form, dihydrotestosterone (DHT), in the prostate.

Researchers made two observations that led them to believe that inhibiting the enzyme and thereby reducing the amount of DHT in the prostate might affect prostate cancer. The first was that male hormones such as DHT seem to feed prostate cancer. The second was that men with a genetic defect that leads to a 5-alpha-reductase deficiency are not troubled by BPH or prostate cancer.

These observations were tested beginning in 1993, when doctors and hospitals across the nation recruited 18,882 healthy men aged 55 and older, and randomized them to receive finasteride (5 mg daily) or a placebo for seven years in an NCI-sponsored study called the Prostate Cancer Prevention Trial. But the trial did not last seven years – it was stopped nearly a year and a half early when independent monitors had enough data to conclude that finasteride had caused a nearly 25 percent reduction in the incidence of prostate cancer in the group. By shrinking prostate size by nearly 25 percent, the drug also reduced the number of urinary problems that might be expected in men 55 and older.

However, there was a glitch: While the drug reduced the incidence of Gleason sum 6 tumors that might be expected in these men, it had no effect on the incidence of Gleason sum 7 tumors and appeared to increase slightly the number of Gleason sum 8 to 10 tumors. The significance of this finding has come into question, and it is likely that many of the high grade cancers were not caused by finasteride, but were found more easily because finasteride not only shrinks the prostate but also makes PSA work better as a screening test, leading to earlier biopsies. Because of this, there is a split in opinion among experts about whether or not it is safe to take finasteride to prevent prostate cancer. The issue may become clearer as more information from this study becomes available.

A compound potent enough to affect the size of a major organ is going to have side effects. Among finasteride's side effects are reduced sexual drive, erectile dysfunction, and ejaculation disorders (primarily decreased volume of ejaculate). These symptoms were also common in the placebo arm of the trial and appeared in fewer than 2 percent of the men taking the drug. In addition, 5-alpha reductase inhibitors have a curious side effect: They grow hair in many men with male-pattern baldness. Not unexpectedly, few men complained about this side effect.

SELENIUM

Selenium, a trace element found in food and soil, is a versatile element used in electronics, photocopy operations, and the manufacture of glass, chemicals, and drugs. It is also a fungicide and feed additive for livestock, particularly horses. Humans get selenium from grains, fish, meat, poultry, eggs, and dairy products. Selenium travels from the soil to plants to animals to humans.

Larry C. Clark, Ph.D., M.P.H., an epidemiologist at the Arizona Cancer Center in Tucson, Arizona, noticed that the incidence of skin cancer varied around the United States and appeared to correlate with selenium levels in the soil. (There is a great deal of variation in the amount of selenium in the soil; it is higher in some geographic regions than in others.) Dr. Clark wondered whether supplementing people's diets with selenium might reduce the incidence of the cancer.

In 1983, he and a coalition of seven dermatology clinics in the Southeastern United States began a study in more than 1,300 men and women to see whether selenium supplements had an effect on basal cell or squamous (scaly) cell skin cancers. The Southeast was chosen because the soil and, consequently, the food it produced had very low levels of the element. Seven years after the trial started, new "secondary" endpoints were added.

The 1990 endpoints included assessment of the incidence of lung, prostate, and colorectal cancers. When the researchers analyzed their data, they were surprised. It looked as if selenium had reduced deaths

ENDPOINTS: NOT THE END

The term "endpoint" can be confusing. In medical studies, it is not necessarily an end but more like a mile marker at which a specific quality is evaluated. For example, the number of prostate cancers appearing after five years in a group taking selenium might be compared to the number of cancers in a group taking a placebo. The study might continue for 15 years, with "endpoints" being reported all along the way.

from cancer by more than half and deaths from prostate cancer by two-thirds. The incidence of colorectal and lung cancer was also cut by half. Ironically, in the long term, selenium actually increased the risk of skin cancer by 14 percent.

These findings surprised the entire medical community. An inexpensive and common dietary supplement that cut the risk of several cancers by half or more was almost too good to be true. The researchers knew they had to double-check their information.

Researchers are now doing just that. In the largest prostate cancer prevention study ever attempted, physicians and medical specialists at 435 sites in the United States, Puerto Rico, and Canada have enrolled 35,534 men, ages 50 and older. The SELECT study – Selenium and Vitamin E Cancer Prevention Trial – will also examine the role Vitamin E may play in cancer prevention.

A word of caution to those individuals who have already decided that selenium is a protective agent and are now taking supplements. The men in the initial Arizona study were taking selenium supplements of 200 mg a day. The National Academy of Sciences believes this is the upper limit of what can be considered safe. The recommended supplement is 55 mcg daily. Levels around 1,000 mcg (1 milligram) can cause gastrointestinal problems and hair and fingernail loss. In addition, the problem with self-administration of supplements such as selenium is that an individual does not know how much dietary selenium might already be in his blood.

VITAMIN E

Vitamin E is a family of natural compounds that dissolve in fats such as the lipids, which are major components of cell membranes. The most active form of the vitamin is alpha-tocopherol, a powerful antioxidant. Vitamin E and the nutrient beta-carotene (found in carrots and sweet potatoes) are others.

Cells burn energy and release waste products in the form of oxygen-free radicals. These atoms or compounds are unbalanced because they lack at least one electron that should be orbiting a nucleus. These atoms seeks balance by stealing electrons wherever they can be found. Free radicals can cause considerable cellular damage; antioxidants such as vitamin E limit the damage by sweeping up the radicals. There is also a good chance that vitamin E is involved in other cellular and hormonal processes.

Strong evidence for alpha-tocopheral's ability to reduce the risk of prostate cancer comes from Finland. Finnish men are heavy smokers and suffer a high incidence of lung cancer. The Finns wanted to find out whether antioxidants such as alpha-tocopheral and beta-carotene (vitamin A) would reduce the incidence of lung cancer. They initiated the ATBC (alpha-tocopherol, beta-carotene cancer prevention) Trial. When the researchers began analyzing the findings about eight years after the trial had started, they found that men taking vitamin E had reduced their risk of prostate cancer by 32 percent. But they also found that vitamin E may not be everyone's supplement of choice because there was a 50 percent increase in deaths from stroke in men with hypertension. And men taking beta-carotene suffered an 18 percent increase in lung cancers and an 8 percent increase in their overall death rate.

One of the more important and often overlooked messages coming out of the data is that you cannot assume that a supplement such as vitamin E or vitamin A is good for you just because it is "natural" or common. If a substance is potent enough to produce good effects in one place, it may be strong enough to cause damage in another.

A second and equally important message is that when you are considering making changes in diet or lifestyle, you must consider the whole lifestyle. Recent data on vitamin E suggest that doses of greater than 400 mg may increase the risk of congestive heart failure in those with underlying risk factors (high blood pressure, known cardiac disease, and diabetes). So before you start taking vitamin E, it is best to discuss your specific risks with your doctor.

SOY

Researchers have wondered why the incidence of prostate cancer among Asians is so much lower than it is among Westerners such as Americans. They reasoned that it could not be genetic, because Japanese men have a low rate of prostate cancer, yet their children and grandchildren living in the United States have a cancer rate similar to their Caucasian and African American neighbors. Were there environmentally related factors? Was it diet?

Soy and soy products such as tofu constitute a major aspect of the Japanese diet. Soybeans are legumes, a family of plants that includes a variety of other beans, peas, peanuts, and lentils. But soybeans are unique in that they are a concentrated source of isoflavones, compounds that behave somewhat like the hormone estrogen when they are eaten. Laboratory studies of isoflavones such as genistein, daidzein, and others show that they can inhibit benign and malignant cell growth, slow down the activity of androgen-regulated genes, and slow tumor growth in animals.

A number of epidemiological studies suggest that soy and soy products (which contain isoflavones) reduce the risk of prostate cancer. One study conducted on 12,395 male Seventh-Day Adventists in California involved soy milk. Seventh-day Adventists have strict dietary regulations, leading many of them to avoid animal products and substitute soy milk for cow milk. The study found that those who drank more than one cup of soy milk a day reduced their risk of prostate cancer by 70 percent.

The study suggests that soy reduces the risk of prostate cancer. But emphasis must be placed on the word "suggest." These and other studies do not *prove* that soy and its isoflavones reduce the incidence of prostate cancer. Remember this when you see advertisements stating that soy and soy products "prevent" prostate and other cancers.

LYCOPENE

This chapter began by noting that a diet rich in pizza was said to reduce the risk of getting prostate cancer. But the effect didn't come from the pizza, it came from the tomato sauce.

It is thought by many that lycopene, a potent antioxidant, is the compound in tomatoes producing the protective effects, but as yet no one can say that with certainty. Small problems crop up. Rats fed tomato powder were protected from prostate cancer. Rats fed pure lycopene were not.

Experiments like this suggest that there may be something else in tomatoes that works with or without lycopene to reduce prostate cancer.

It was noted earlier that tomato juice had little if any protective effect, whereas tomatoes cooked lightly in oil did. Did the cooking alter the chemical makeup of the tomatoes? Or were there other compounds in the final preparation? These are unanswered questions. There have been a few small studies of lycopene in men who had already been diagnosed with prostate cancer. They were put on a lycopene-based diet regimen for about three weeks before they underwent radical prostatectomy. In both studies, the diet appeared to reduce the size of the prostate and lower PSA. But the differences were slight and the studies were too small to allow firm conclusions.

GREEN TEA

This tea, another staple of the Asian diet, contains polyphenols, compounds with antioxidant properties that give the tea its "tang" or astringency. The idea that green tea may offer a degree of protection against prostate cancer is derived as a general idea from epidemiology studies of Asian diets. Laboratory scientists have taken a closer look at the polyphenols in green tea in a number of animal experiments and report that the polyphenols slow the growth of prostate cancer cells in mice and seem to inhibit several oncogenes, the genes that cause cancer. Nothing has yet been proven in human beings. Headlines that proclaim "Green Tea Prevents Cancer" are premature.

COX-2 INHIBITORS

When the body's normal biological processes are disrupted by injury or a disease such as cancer, the defense system is turned on and the inflammatory response kicks in. One of the products of a long chain of inflammatory actions is cyclooxegenase 2 (COX-2), an enzyme that influences the production of prostaglandin. The prostaglandin produced in response to COX-2 activity can encourage tumor formation, the proliferation of new cells, and the development of blood vessels that eventually feed tumors and growing cells. Researchers have found that prostate cancer cells produce more COX-2 than normal prostate cells. They also found that COX-2 production can be

Researchers found that COX-2 production can be limited by nonsteroidal anti-inflammatory drugs (NSAIDS), also known as COX-2 inhibitors.

limited by nonsteroidal anti-inflammatory drugs (NSAIDS), also known as COX-2 inhibitors. Some of the more familiar NSAIDS are aspirin, ibuprofen, indomethacin, and naproxen.

Inhibiting COX-2 production significantly slows the growth of prostate cancer cell lines. Adding vitamin D to the NSAIDS has a synergistic effect. (This is an effect in which the results are stronger than one would expect by adding the benefits of one drug or substance to the benefits of another.) These are experiments conducted in test tubes and petri dishes. The results have yet to be proven in animals, much less humans. A clinical trial that might have shed some light on the question was stopped when it was shown that the NSAID involved, rofecoxib (Vioxx), was associated with heart attacks and strokes.

RED WINE

Red wine is a rich source of phytochemicals; some of these chemical compounds are polyphenols such as catechins and resveratrol, which are thought to have antioxidant or anti-cancer properties.

Polyphenols are antioxidant compounds found in the skin and seeds of grapes. When wine is made from grapes, the alcohol produced by the fermentation process dissolves the polyphenols contained in the skin and seeds. Red wine contains more polyphenols than white wine because grape skins are removed during the making of white wine.

Research on the antioxidants found in red wine has shown that they may help inhibit the development of certain cancers, although polyphenols have not been directly tested for prostate cancer.

CHALLENGE AND CHOICE

If you are old enough to become concerned about prostate cancer or if, like Dave, you are old enough to have been diagnosed with the disease, you are old enough to start living a life that's a little healthier. Age, at this point, is a double-edged sword. You are old enough to be smart, yet you are old enough to have settled into some longstanding habits, some of which may be hard to break. Straightening out and replacing those habits with newer, healthier ones can be tough, but it can be done.

Staying healthy and fighting disease is hard work. There are no shortcuts. When you begin exploring the literature on prostate cancer on the Internet (see Appendix), you will find plenty of handy information. You will also encounter websites touting supplements, many with claims that border on the ridiculous. Get your information from well-established sources such as nationally recognized associations, institutions, and medical publications that are produced by honest health-care specialists. And no matter what information you acquire, talk to your doctor about it. ◆

Chapter 8

Clinical Trials

When confronted with a disease, one has a natural inclination to want to understand as much as possible about the disease and its associated treatments.

Dave is now learning everything there is about prostate cancer and its treatment. He dives into books, magazines, and the Internet in search of the latest medicines and therapeutic innovations, and finds thousands of pages of health-related literature available at the tap of a few computer keys. Some of it is worthwhile. Much of it is confusing, misleading, or outright wrong.

A few years ago, the only source of reliable information about a specific disease was the public library. The library remains an excellent source of fundamental information about health care, but the advent of the Internet and the proliferation of computers render inadequate all other means of acquiring the most recent medical information. This is the information jungle. At one extreme, there are medical publications and websites that present the most advanced scientific ideas and medical information. At the other end, there are the hucksters' sites that describe new therapies in terms so glowing as to lead one to suspect their veracity. One should explore these sites with an open mind, yet be suspicious if something sounds too good to be true.

SEARCHING THE WEB

When wandering the Internet, it is wise to stick to safe neighborhoods. Well-known institutions and recognized organizations provide detailed and sound information on specific diseases. The National Cancer Institute (www.cancer.gov), the American Cancer

Society (www.cancer.org), and the Prostate Cancer Foundation (www.prostatecancerfoundation.org) are great places to start a quest. Nationally recognized institutions such as Cleveland Clinic (www.clevelandclinic.org) offer valuable information on specific diseases and treatments. In addition, these sites usually link to other Internet sites that are home to support groups such as the American Foundation for Urologic Disease (www.afud.org), another good source of information. Your physician should also be able to provide you with the URLs of Internet support groups, such as www.ustoo.com, www.malecare.com, and www.yananow.net, to name a few, as well as the names of local support groups.

One of the primary functions of these institutions and support groups is to keep interested people informed about the most recent developments in the field. The news that the media and proprietary websites offer is invariably secondhand information – reports of articles published in medical journals. If you are truly interested in a specific aspect of a disease or a new therapy, you are going to have to go to the source – the clinical study.

READING CLINICAL STUDIES

Reading these pages is not as intimidating as they first may seem. Every medical study in the literature follows a fundamental format consisting of an abstract, introduction, protocol, materials and methods, results, discussion, and conclusion. Here's what those terms mean:

Abstract. The abstract is a condensed version of the article. It will tell you why the study was conducted, what animals or patients (and how many) were involved, how they were treated, what the researchers found, and what the researchers think of what they found. Abstracts are presented so that readers do not have to wade through thousands of words. Basically, the abstract will tell you whether the article has information that is appropriate for your situation and whether it is of interest to you.

Introduction. Here the researchers, often appropriately called investigators, explain why they initiated the study and the potential effect its outcome might have. They note how many people suffer from the disease, what the limitations of current therapies might be, and why a new therapy or a new way of delivering an existing therapy shows promise. Then they state the question they hope the ensuing study will answer.

Protocol. The protocol is the design of the study. It spells out what sorts of people were selected to participate in the trial and how the medications or treatments were administered. This section of the study should be read carefully, for it will show how closely the study reflects the clinical situation in which you might be interested.

Materials and methods. This is invariably a dense description of exactly how the study was conducted, including the tools that were used (right down to makes and models) and whether medicines were delivered in the morning or evening. The methods section is detailed for several reasons. Medical studies are published in juried or peer-reviewed journals. That means that before the study gets into print, the manuscript is reviewed by specialists in the field who look for flaws or mistakes in the way the study was conducted. They read the paper and respond with observations about the quality of the work, and they often have a number of questions for the authors, such as "Why did you use one drug and not another?" And "Can you explain in greater detail the nature of the side effects?"

It is difficult to get a medical study into print, especially in a prestigious journal. Often, the news media and lay journals will describe the findings of studies that are reported at meetings before they are published. Such stories should be carefully scrutinized. If the findings reported at the annual meeting of the American Urological Association, the American Association for Cancer Research, the American Society of Clinical Oncology, or any other such group are accurate and important, the research will eventually make its way to a peer-reviewed journal. If the findings are very important, they will appear in such journals pretty quickly. If the study is never heard of again, there is a reason.

Results. This is another section that is dense with detail and data. It contains the details of the findings, often in numerical or graphic format, and details on the statistical methods used to justify the article's conclusion. Unless you have a background in statistics or mathematics, this section may be hard to understand.

Discussion. The authors of the paper will state what was unusual, surprising, or promising about the information.

Conclusion. The authors will restate what they think was important about their study, what they believe the study's most significant findings are, and what the next step should be.

HOW DO NEW THERAPIES EVOLVE?

Therapies begin as research; they arrive in pharmacies only at the end of Phase III drug or research trials. Very few treatment breakthroughs complete this very long journey.

It is worthwhile to mark a treatment's location along the route. There are many hurdles to overcome before a drug can be considered for use in humans. The hierarchy of tests a drug must pass is as follows: in vitro studies, in vivo studies, Phase I trials, Phase II trials, Phase III trials, and Phase IV studies.

In vitro. This is Latin for "in a glass." These are very fundamental studies. Every so often, the media will report a striking advance against cancer only to reveal in the fifth paragraph that the cancer was stopped in a petri dish. In vitro studies form the foundation of all future experiments, but they are simple, isolated laboratory environments. A drug that acts against a cancer cell line in a dish or test tube may lose its effectiveness completely when it encounters the thousands upon thousands of differing proteins and compounds found in a living vessel.

In vivo. This is Latin for "in life." These are studies conducted in living organisms beginning with the simplest and moving to the more complex. Many are conducted in "animal models." These are animals whose immune systems or organs have been modified to allow the diseases they harbor to mimic the diseases that human beings suffer.

Studies conducted in test tubes and animals are experimental studies. Studies conducted in humans are called clinical trials.

Phase I trials. These trials involve a small number of patients and are often conducted in individuals who are perfectly healthy. Their intent is to evaluate a therapy's safety, to identify side effects, and (when drugs and/or radiation treatment is involved) to determine a safe, though not necessarily optimal dosage. Sometimes, they are called "dose-ranging" trials.

For example, in August 2006, Mt. Sinai Medical Center in New York was conducting a Phase I trial involving gene therapy to control tumor growth in prostate cancer patients. And a joint study involving the Indiana University Cancer Center and Long Island College Hospital is investigating the use of ultrasound energy to see whether it can kill cancer cells without affecting the surrounding tissue. These are just a few examples of some of the fascinating research projects being conducted around the country.

Phase II trials. These trials are conducted in a larger body of patients. The researchers are trying to find out what the maximally tolerated dose is for further testing in Phase III trials. A secondary goal is to get an inkling of whether the therapy actually works and whether it produces better results than existing therapies.

One intriguing Phase II trial conducted at Duke University's Comprehensive Cancer Center in August 2006 involved exercise and dietary counseling, and how they may improve physical activity, nutrition, and quality of life in older long-term cancer survivors who are overweight.

Phase III trials. These trials can involve hundreds to thousands of people. By this time, the researchers believe the new therapy works better than existing therapies, or just as well but with fewer and less severe side effects. Phase III testing will help determine with a degree of precision how well the drug works, compared to placebo or an existing treatment; how well it works in some people; and how ineffective it may be for others.

One study at Wake Forest University that reached the Phase III level in August 2006 involves using soy protein, isoflavones, and venlafaxine to treat hot flashes in prostate cancer patients receiving hormone therapy. A similar study underway at the Sidney Kimmel Comprehensive Cancer Center at Johns Hopkins University has reached the Phase IV level. And here at Cleveland Clinic, we're investigating whether Reiki energy healing affects disease progression and anxiety in patients with localized prostate cancer who are candidates for radical prostatectomy.

Phase IV trials. These are conducted to gather information after a drug has been approved. These studies involve significant numbers of patients and reveal with greater accuracy how well the drug works in specific clinical situations and how frequently side effects appear in specific groups of patients.

STUDY AND TRIAL DESIGN

A trial's design is important, for it can affect the strength or certainty of the conclusions that are made when the final data sets are analyzed. Trials may be *prospective* or *retrospective*. A prospective study is designed to follow participants forward in time and uses carefully defined protocols to determine an outcome that is unknown beforehand. In retrospective studies, investigators sift through clinical records and other available medical evidence seeking insights that those who initially recorded the data may not have sought. In other words, in prospective trials, the questions are asked first, and the trial is designed to answer them; in retrospective studies, the data are collected and then questions are asked.

For example, investigators may retrospectively review the records of all patients treated for Gleason sum 6 cancer during the past 10 years to see whether overweight men were more likely to experience recurrent cancer than men with normal body weight. They might compare the recurrence rates of radiation therapy in overweight men to recurrence rates of overweight prostatectomy patients. These studies frequently produce insights, but they have a weakness. That is, because the initial trial was not specifically designed to answer the questions now being asked, the data needed to answer them may be incomplete or inaccurately recorded.

In addition, trials are either *selected* or *randomized.* Selected trials involve patients and treatments that are carefully selected in order to get optimal results from a treatment or to find out how a treatment performs in specific clinical situations. Phase I and II trials, designed to test the effectiveness of a drug and identify its side effects, are often selected trials. But in the real world, no two clinical situations are the same. This is why randomized Phase III trials are thought to produce findings that will have the greatest value in the clinic. Flipping a coin to determine which patients get one treatment and which patients get another treatment is as good a means as any to randomize a group of patients.

Trials are either *blinded* or *open.* Blinded trials are thought to produce findings similar to those in the real world, and double-blind trials produce the best data. In a blinded trial, patients do not know whether they are getting an active drug or a placebo, or which of two active treatments they are getting. Patients who think they are getting medication will sometimes improve even though the medication is no more than a sugar pill. This is known as a placebo effect. It is a powerful effect that can complicate many trials, especially smaller ones. In double-blinded trials, neither the patient nor the treating physician knows who is getting medication and who is getting placebo. This is because physicians are as prone to bias as patients, and if they think a patient is getting a good treatment, they will see improvements or encourage the patient to report improvements.

> In a blinded trial, patients do not know whether they are getting an active drug or a placebo, or which of two active treatments they are getting.

The "gold standard" of trials then is a prospective, randomized, double-blinded trial involving a large number of patients, usually hundreds if not thousands.

DECIPHERING MEDICAL LINGO

There is an extensive vocabulary associated with medical reporting. Defining all the terms would fill a pocket dictionary, but there are some terms that should be known to prevent a misreading of clinical studies and reports.

Arm. Patients in studies are placed in groups called arms. There is a treatment arm, a placebo arm, a treatment plus counseling arm, and so forth.

Cohort. The difference between a cohort and an arm is that a cohort can exist within an arm. A cohort usually is a group that shares a specific quality. For instance, a study arm might be broken into a cohort of younger men receiving treatment vs. a cohort of older men receiving treatment, or thin men vs. obese men. This is done to determine which patients are most likely to get the greatest benefit from a therapy. It is also done to unearth factors that influence the treatment. A cohort of men taking vitamin E supplements may do better with a certain treatment than men who are not. This would suggest that vitamin E is somehow working with the drug to produce better results, a finding that will no doubt lead to a recommendation to include vitamin E in the treatment regimen.

Control group. This is the foundation group against which the treatment group is compared. These might be men receiving no treatment, or men with the disease being treated with what is currently considered "standard" therapy. Some studies will include a control group, a placebo arm, and a treatment group.

Treatment group. These are the patients getting the treatment the study is investigating.

Significance. This term is often misunderstood or misinterpreted by laymen. It does not mean that the study's findings constitute a major advance. A finding is said to be "statistically significant" when the difference between the control group and the treatment group was likely to be caused by the treatment and not chance, the placebo effect, or bias.

Statements will be made to the effect that "40 percent of the treatment group showed improvement as compared to 37 percent of the control group. The results were statistically significant." A 3 percent difference may not seem like big deal, but because it achieved "statistical significance," it shows that the treatment actually had some effect. This might not be sufficient to get the treatment approved, but it may be sufficient to cause researchers to continue trying to improve the treatment.

P-value. When a research paper states a treatment is statistically significant, it will often append a "P-value," as in "40 percent of the treatment group showed improvement as compared to 37 percent of the control group. The results were statistically significant. (P = 0.002)"

The P-value shows how strong the significance of a finding might be and how likely the difference between two groups is to be true, rather than the result of random chance. It is generally accepted that in order for findings to achieve significance, they must have a P-value of at least 0.05 or lower. At the level of P = 0.05 there is a 1 in 20 possibility that the difference between treatment and placebo is the result of chance or bias. At P = 0.005, the odds that the difference is purely chance are 1 in 200.

Confidence interval. This is a measure of the accuracy of data being reported. "Some 82 percent of men reported improvement (95% CI = 82 - 92)." That means that there is a 95 percent chance that if the study were conducted again, the results would fall between 82 percent and 92 percent. Most studies report data at the 95 percent confidence level, although some go higher.

Odds ratio. The odds ratio is the chance of something happening in a group being studied as compared to a control group. For instance, the control group is men who do not take a new type of natural supplement (Group A). The study group (Group B) takes the supplement once a day. At the end of five years, it is found that Group B has 9 percent fewer cancers than Group A. The odds ratio for Group B is therefore 0.91. If Group B has 9 percent more cancers than Group A, the odds ratio would be 1.09.

GETTING INVOLVED

There are several reasons to consider joining a clinical trial. It provides a chance to become more actively involved in your own care. Trials offer access to advanced treatments. There is a caveat: In many trials, participants have only a 50-50 chance of getting the active or new medication; some get the placebo. Still, participating in a trial is an opportunity to contribute to advancing research and possibly to provide future generations with the benefits of a new therapy.

Finding a prostate cancer trial is not hard. The National Cancer Institute's web page is the best place to start looking. On June 15, 2007, the NCI listed 380 different prostate cancer trials that were under way or enrolling patients. (Go to www.cancer.gov for more information.)

The NCI web page is a tribute to advancing technology. In a few minutes, you can acquire information that would have once taken days to discover. The page allows you to search for clinical trials by stage (stage I, II, III), by character (treatment trials, supportive care trial, screening trials, prevention trials, and diagnostic trials), and by proximity – trials within 20, 50, 100, or 200 miles of your home.

Once you visit www.cancer.gov, click on the "Clinical Trials" bar at the top of the page. Enter the relevant information – type of cancer, type of trial, and location (how far you would be willing to travel to participate in a study). Once you do that, you will get a description of the trial, its purpose and eligibility criteria, and trial contact information.

This is only information. Getting involved with a trial requires more effort than clicking a mouse. Patients joining trials are rigorously screened to determine their eligibility and to identify the parameters of their health or illness to ensure that when the trial's data are analyzed later, the findings will be reasonably accurate. The trial's designers want P to be greater than 0.05.

Screening includes an "informed consent" process. This is a consultation with a trial representative whose job is to make sure that the potential enrollee understands every aspect of the trial, including known risks and what is being expected of him. Enrollees must think of themselves as participants, not patients. Many trials require enrollees to adhere to a rigorous lifestyle and keep careful records of their health in order to identify treatment effects and side effects.

Trials are not for those who are merely sick. Trials are for those who are sick and want to do something about it. They are work.

TALK TO YOUR PHYSICIAN

Prostate cancer is the most common cancer men suffer and, as bizarre as it may seem, that is a substantial benefit. It means that there is a major research effort under way to develop new therapies. Getting information is not the problem: Type "prostate cancer" into the Google search engine and you will get more than 25 million responses. The challenge for patients and their families is to sort the good information from the bad, and there is plenty of bad. It is a good idea to understand as much as you can about the disease. It is a better idea to discuss everything you learn with your physician. Curiously, one of the more important roles physicians play is that of "myth buster." ◆

Chapter 9

Research

*The most exciting phrase to hear in science,
the one that heralds the new discoveries, is not "Eureka!"
["I found it!"] but "That's funny ..."*

– Isaac Asimov

Many people that Dave will never meet are working on solving his prostate problem. He will never know how many, and we are unable to tell him because the full scope of prostate cancer research is impossible to quantify. In the United States alone, thousands of skilled, dedicated, and determined men and women are working on learning as much as possible about Dave's type of cancer and its treatment.

The U.S. government spends about $485 million annually for prostate cancer research, but this is only a portion of the total being spent on all types of research. The figure does not reflect the contributions made by foundations, institutions, or even individuals. The research projects range from a single physician examining data from a series of surgeries he has performed to "multi-center" studies involving dozens of health-care institutions around the globe.

In light of the breadth of this effort, it is impossible to describe all the research now underway. And it would be foolish to try to identify which projects might yield the most startling advance. When experts label a research initiative "promising," what many of them mean is that it hasn't failed yet. Hundreds of new therapies clear one hurdle after another, only to fall by the wayside when it is found that the treatment's adverse side effects outweigh the benefits, or that the results achieved are not as good as those of treatments that are already well established. The so-called "breakthroughs" make news maybe once a decade or less. Failures just go away.

The National Cancer Institute segregates its research funding into eight categories:

- Treatment
- Prevention
- Early detection to include diagnosis and prognosis
- Cancer control to include survivorship and outcomes research
- Biology
- Causes
- Biologic models
- Other projects

The following paragraphs describe some of the research being conducted in each of these categories. The experiments and studies were selected not because they are particularly promising, but because they exemplify the nature of the research, the mysteries investigators must resolve, the tools they use, the progress they are making, and the ingenuity they often employ to try to understand the disease. This research also demonstrates the complexity of cancer and the challenge these scientists, specialists, and health-care workers face when trying to defeat cancer.

TREATMENT

Here's one project now being worked on: Investigators at many institutions are studying a number of signal transduction agents, which are communication systems that are involved in the growth and metastasis (spread) of cancer cells. Hormones influence the cancerous processes. Hormones are in constant circulation, but they affect only cells that display specific hormone receptors on their surfaces.

Like a piece of a jigsaw puzzle, every molecule has a specific shape. For the hormone to have any effect, its shape must fit perfectly into the shape receptor on the surface of the cell. This prompts a cascade of signals – like the numbers that open a safe – that cross the cell membrane and interior of the cell to eventually reach the DNA in the cell's nucleus. Genes in the DNA are switched on or off to influence the cell's cycle of life, division, and death.

In the signal that transduction agents project, researchers want to identify specific molecules that influence specific genes. If a cancerous cell were a clock, these people would be taking it apart to see what makes it tick. But a cancerous cell is not a clock – it has far more parts and is much smaller. An understanding of the signaling mechanisms that relay hormonal messages from the outer membrane to the nucleus and back would allow drugs to be designed that either amplify or block the signals and therefore halt the cancer's growth.

Other researchers are studying a new technology known as "magnetic resonance spectroscopic imaging" (MRSI), which offers an image of the chemical makeup of the prostate. The benefit of this new process is that it will show physicians where the cancer cells are growing. Cancer cells tend to metabolize (burn) more citrate – a citric acid – than normal cells. Investigators think that if they can accurately locate tiny areas where citrate is being burned, they can more accurately insert radioactive seeds or other therapeutic agents into probable tumors and destroy them. They also think MRSI will tell them how well these therapies have worked after the seeds have been implanted.

PREVENTION

The following two research projects show that researchers are willing to look anywhere and everywhere for new therapies, from the bottom of Chinese teacups to the paint on the faces of American Indians. Sometimes it seems that if there is even the slightest hint that a substance might have beneficial effects, a scientist somewhere is going to check it out.

Epidemiologists have shown that Asian men have less prostate cancer than Caucasian men and that one of the reasons for this may be that they drink lots of green tea. Laboratory researchers have found that substances in green tea known as catechins inhibit the growth of prostate cancer cell lines in test tubes, and they also inhibit the cell's ability to secrete substances that promote angiogenesis, the growth of new blood vessels. (Tumors need sustenance to grow. To acquire sustenance, they secrete substances that promote the development of new blood vessels that will bring them the food they need.)

> **Laboratory researchers have found that substances in green tea known as catechins inhibit the growth of prostate cancer cell lines in test tubes.**

One of the green tea catechins, a substance labeled (-)-epigallocatechin-3-gallate (EGCG), is particularly good at inhibiting cell growth and angiogenesis. A group in Texas is taking a close look at this. The researchers hypothesize that EGCG works by preventing cells from making the factors that promote angiogenesis, thereby starving growing tumors.

And a group in Wisconsin is taking a close look at *Sanguinaria canadensis,* more commonly known as bloodroot. It is a small flowering plant whose petals open in the spring throughout the woods of Midwestern North America. Native Americans used it as body paint and spread it on sores, warts, and other skin problems. They also ingested it in small doses as a stimulant like coffee and in large doses to induce vomiting.

Researchers want to find out what effect sanguinarine, a substance derived from the plant's root, will have on various prostate cancer cell lines. This means more than putting a little sanguinarine in a dish with cancer cells and watching what happens. The work involves extensive molecular studies to identify the specific cellular machinery that is affected by the substance. Unfortunately, while the research is being conducted, unscrupulous so-called herbal healers are using the Internet to tout bloodroot as a "cure" for cancer. The FDA considers bloodroot to be toxic and unsafe, but since the alleged remedy is "natural" rather than manufactured, there is little that can be done to prevent its sale.

EARLY DETECTION, DIAGNOSIS, AND PROGNOSIS

The "gray range" of PSA values, the region from 4 ng/mL to 10 ng/mL, troubles everyone. Readings that fall into this range suggest that the next step should be a biopsy, but about 75 percent of the biopsies conducted in this range turn up negative. Many people are looking for ways to more accurately identify the presence of cancer.

Think of the California Gold Rush, when prospectors squatted on their haunches beside a stream and washed water across silt to try to find gold. Today, scientists wash serum samples across microarrays. The common components of the serum wash away; what sticks are the proteins that may help identify a disease such as cancer.

Our immune system identifies cancer tissue as unusual and produces antibodies to the proteins. These are called antigens. Some antigens are associated with cancer; some are not. Those antigens that only bind to cancer-related antigens are called autoantibodies.

So, when a patient's serum is washed across the microarray, autoantibodies in the serum will stick to the antigens in the "pan" while the rest will wash away. The resulting pattern in the tray (called an "autoantibody signature") is the fingerprint of cancer – at least, researchers in Michigan hope it will turn out that way. They have been working on a test that they hope will supplement the PSA test and reduce the troubling number of false positives produced by the PSA screen. This would eliminate a substantial number of unnecessary biopsies and the cost and inconvenience associated with them. By identifying proteins associated with the cancer, the technology also has the potential to tell us much more about the character of the disease than we now know.

Researchers at a number of institutions are looking at assays that measure levels of human kallikrein 2 (hK2), a compound that resembles PSA and is produced in prostate cells, particularly prostate cancer cells. Work is being done to develop tests that will determine how much hK2 is being produced in normal states, as compared to cancerous states. The idea is that if levels of hK2 can be juxtaposed against levels of PSA in a mathematical formula, the results will be a test that more accurately predicts prostate cancer in men whose PSA is below 10 ng/mL. This is not easy. The challenge is not only to find needles in a haystack, but also to determine exactly how many needles there are for every bushel of hay in the stack.

CANCER CONTROL, SURVIVORSHIP, AND OUTCOMES RESEARCH

Investigators in Washington, D.C., are trying to create the optimal educational brochure: One that will answer all the questions a man might have about prostate cancer and give him the tools for making informed decisions about getting screened.

To do this, researchers are offering free screenings. When men call to register for the screening, they will be randomized to four different groups:

- Men given both basic and more detailed information one week before screening
- Men given only basic information a week before screening
- Men given most packets of information the day of screening
- Men given only basic information on the day of screening

The investigators then intend to track these men for a year to see how they responded to the information and the timing of its delivery. Putting together a brochure may seem like no big deal, but if the research team creates an effective way of getting men to set up appointments for exams, they could save as many lives as any new therapy.

Another study being conducted in Brooklyn shows how imaginative scientists can be when trying to reach people. This group is hanging out at barbershops to observe how barbers communicate with customers. Then they intend to give those same barbers an education on prostate cancer and the benefits of examinations, hoping they will pass the information along to their customers.

BIOLOGY

At one time, the best a physician could do was to hand a patient some medication and say, "Take this and tell me what happens." With today's technology, scientists know what certain medications do to specific molecules and genes inside a single cell. Researchers can sift through thousands of proteins the way archaeologists sift sand for pottery shards, find the ones they think are important, and then begin to manage them.

A group in California is looking closely at one of these shards – a protein factor dubbed "early growth response-1" (Egr-1). It seems that prostate cancer cells produce much more of this factor than do normal cells. The researchers also have found that in animals, tumors that do not have a great deal of Egr-1 tend to remain stable rather than metastasize. This is prompting a very close look at Egr-1. If the factor is found to be important for growth and metastasis, the next step is to develop an agent that blocks its effects.

When a gene in a cell's DNA is turned on, it produces messenger RNA (mRNA), a strand of amino acids that is a coded message telling the cell's machinery what proteins should be made. If a cell is producing Egr-1, there must be an mRNA strand holding the coded message for that factor. The scientists hope to decipher the mRNA code and build a strand of antisense RNA, a specific "monkey-wrench" that will gum up a specific piece of cellular machinery.

Antisense RNA is something like a reflection of the primary mRNA in a mirror. It is an exact opposite. As an opposite, it will stick to the primary mRNA and prevent it from delivering the message. No message, no Egr-1. No Egr-1, no tumor growth or metastasis. That is the goal.

One of the important ideas to draw from studies like this and others is that scientists now have the ability to do what cells do. They can design specific molecules that will have specific functions. It should also be noted that science cannot do it as well or as efficiently as cells can, but that issue is being worked on.

Whereas metastatic cancer cells appear to make more Egr-1 than normal cells, it also appears that they produce less Raf kinase inhibitor protein (RKIP). If the gene that produces Egr-1 can be considered a tumor *promoter* gene, then the RKIP gene is considered a tumor suppressor gene. Turning off a tumor-suppressor gene is like releasing the handbrake of a truck parked on a hill. Researchers in the Michigan lab that is developing the microarray are also manipulating levels of RKIP in prostate cancer cell lines to see what happens. They want to figure out how RKIP prevents cancers from becoming metastatic.

CAUSES, ETIOLOGY

Prostate specific membrane antigen (PSMA) is like PSA, but is produced almost exclusively in prostate membrane cells. Prostate cancer cells produce more PSMA than do normal cells, and this action may influence cell growth.

PSMA breaks down folates (vitamin B compounds) and where there is a lot of PSMA, there is a lot of folate being broken down, which seems to change the internal structure of prostate cells. (Researchers call this structure the cell's histologic architecture.) Working with several mouse strains that are particularly susceptible to prostate cancer, researchers intend to block PSMA's folate activity and manipulate the amount of vitamin B in the animals' diets to see what effect blocking the PSMA will have on their propensity to develop cancer.

The study is far more complicated than simply giving mice more vitamin B and seeing what happens. With the tools they now have, researchers intend to find out what vitamin B manipulation does to specific genes. This is another example of seeing what happens when you throw a monkey wrench into the works. These men and women are looking for both the right wrench and the specific works into which it can be jammed.

Some researchers are not at all hesitant about declaring the importance of their work. The International Consortium for Prostate Cancer Genetics (ICPCG) candidly states that its database provides "an unprecedented opportunity to characterize and unravel the complexities of genetic susceptibility for this common disease." It may be right. Prostate cancer has a genetic component. In Dave's case, because he had a first-degree relative with prostate cancer – his father – the chances that he may develop the cancer are significantly increased. The same would have been true if Dave had a brother with prostate cancer. The hereditary form of prostate cancer may account for up to one in 10 or more cancers. The ICPCG, a group of 20 institutions in seven countries, has collected DNA samples from 1,700 prostate cancer families. Hereditary cancer has been associated with genes situated at six different loci.

A word about genetics: A locus is a specific physical location or region of a chromosome. Researchers may or may not know the exact DNA code for a gene, but they can tell where it is located, owing to alterations in the gene's structure. If you compare a normal gene to the same gene taken from someone with hereditary cancer, it is possible that the cancer gene weighs a little more or a little less. This suggests that it has something extra in its makeup. In this instance, the ICPCG is looking at six different loci believed to hold prostate cancer associated genes. One gene or combinations of these genes may carry the risk of hereditary cancer.

Successfully tracking abnormal genes to specific locations on chromosomes offers several unique opportunities. If the genes are shown to be associated with cancer risk, simple genetic tests can be created to allow physicians to assess cancer risk in specific patients. It also lets researchers narrow their search for the genes themselves. Once they have identified the genes, they can begin to understand what the genes make and how that product influences cancer. This is a major step toward developing therapies that either enhance or impede the gene's activity.

Three observations can be derived from the preceding study:

- Some scientific endeavors are simply too big for a single researcher, laboratory, or institution. Even the busiest oncology center would be hard-pressed to get DNA samples from 1,700 families with a history of prostate cancer.

- Most medical progress is made by investigators who share their discoveries. Medical breakthroughs are not the bailiwick of a solitary white-frocked scientist bent over a microscope, poking a cell with a needle and shouting "Eureka!"

- The key ingredients of scientific achievement are diligence and patience.

Team research can often create wonderful effects. Recently, researchers from a consortium of 14 institutions, including the National Human Genome Research Institute, Johns Hopkins Medical Institutions, and Cleveland Clinic have identified a gene on chromosome 1 that shows an association with an inherited form of prostate cancer in some families. The researchers reported an association between mutations in a gene on chromosome 1 called ribonuclease L (RNase L) and an increased risk of developing prostate cancer in men from some families with a history of the disease. The gene encodes a protein, also called RNase L, which functions as an enzyme. Scientists already know that the enzyme protects cells from viral infections and also causes defective cells to die. The new study shows that in men from families with a history of prostate cancer, several different types of mutations can inactivate the RNase L gene, and the inactivation appears to predispose the individual to prostate cancer. Robert Silverman, Ph.D., a cancer biologist at the Cleveland Clinic, was instrumental in this study.

Here is an interesting question: Could cancer be a response to an infection? That question was addressed by a team of researchers from Cleveland Clinic and the University of California, San Francisco, who recently discovered a new virus called XMRV in prostate tumors. Advancing the theory involving RNase L, the group noticed that mice deficient in RNase L were more susceptible to viral infection, and the introduction of RNase L to mouse cells caused cell death to occur. Further, there is evidence in humans that genetic variants of the RNase L may increase their risk of developing prostate cancer. In a study of 150 men, the researchers determined that XMRV is 25 times more likely to be found in prostate cancer patients with a specific genetic predisposition to prostate cancer than it is to be found in men who do not possess the genetic susceptibility.

SCIENTIFIC MODEL SYSTEMS

There are two ways to study prostate cancer in animals. One is to take cancer tissue from a line of cells or other tissue and implant it in an animal. Tissue transplanted from one species to another is called a xenograft. These are common because it is easier to develop a line of cancer cells and implant them than it is to genetically alter an entire animal such as a mouse.

But an animal model offers opportunities for research that xenografts do not. Cancer in a xenograft is already developed. In an animal model, the course of the cancer can be charted from the time it is initiated to the time it reaches its full power. Cancer is a growing organism that changes over time. By taking tissue samples from the animals at regular intervals and analyzing them, researchers can tell what genes are being turned on or off as the cancer progresses.

Investigators in California are not building a better mousetrap. Rather, they are endeavoring to construct a better mouse, one that will allow them to study three specific genes. A gene known as "fibroblast growth factor-8" (FGF-8) is sensitive to male hormones. When the gene is stimulated, cells start to proliferate. Another gene creates retinoid receptors that are thought to have a role in prostate cancer. Retinoids are vitamin A compounds. It has already been shown that vitamin A has an effect on prostate cancer. The Pten (phosphatase and tensin homolog) is a tumor-suppressing gene. When it is turned off, tumor development follows.

Single genes may raise the risk of prostate cancer, but it is doubtful that any single gene causes the disease. Rather, a host of genes acting together in an elaborate dance of give-and-take allows a cancer cell to develop its abnormal characteristics. A mouse model harboring these genes and gene mutations would allow researchers to study these interactions as cancer develops.

Photodynamic therapy is an ingenious new approach to obliterating cancer cells and tumors. The therapy involves the intravenous injection of a photosensitizing (light-sensitive) chemical. This agent is absorbed by cells that are growing at a faster than normal rate. When light of a specific frequency strikes these cells, the agent absorbs the light and produces a form of oxygen (singlet oxygen) that is lethal to the cells. One of the primary advantages of this therapy is that healthy cells, those that did not ingest the photosensitizer, are spared. The disadvantage is that the treatment is limited to surface tumors because the light penetrates only 3 cm (about 1/8th inch) into tissue. It is now used to treat esophageal cancer, lung cancer, and gastric cancers – all tumors that appear on the surface of tissues.

The problem facing those who want to tackle prostate cancer with this new therapy is getting the light to cells deep inside tumors. The solution may lie in inserting light-emitting diodes (LEDs), small semiconductors, into malignant tissue that has absorbed the photosensitizer. This treatment could be seen as something akin to brachytherapy, but it would involve implanting light-emitting diodes instead of radioactive seeds. No two prostates and no two tumors have the same shape. Researchers in Toledo, Ohio, are developing a computer program that will allow the LEDs to be implanted into the prostate so that the cancer-killing light will be evenly distributed throughout cancerous tissue. If they accomplish their goal, they will have a blueprint for applying the therapy not only to prostate cancers but to many other solid tumors as well. ◆

Chapter 10

Moving Forward

The medical advances made during the past 50 years are astounding. Yet it is something of a tribute to the wily cancer cell that despite billions of dollars and insights by the best medical minds, it still manages to evade all attempts at a curative therapy.

Cancer is exceedingly treatable, but we cannot yet say that it can be cured. The risks can be reduced substantially, but the disease cannot yet be totally prevented. Still, when researchers reveal just a little more about how cancerous cells grow or respond to outside interference, they are spurred to even greater efforts.

It would be nice to say that a cure or preventive vaccine is close, but there is really no way of knowing that. However, one statement can be made with certainty: The development of a curative therapy and effective prevention are closer today than they were yesterday, and they will be closer tomorrow than they are today.

The problem Dave has with prostate cancer should not be minimized. It is a big problem, but there are solutions. There is a joke urologists tell each other but seldom tell patients. A doctor walks into the examination room with a clipboard and tells the patient sitting there, "I've got bad news and good news. The bad news is that you have cancer. The good news is that it is prostate cancer."

Dave's cancer will be treated, that's a certainty, and it is likely that he will be cured. And one day he may be standing with a group of his buddies on the third tee of a local golf course when one of them might blurt out, "Well, I guess you guys should know. My doctor thinks I might have prostate cancer."

And if all goes well for Dave and his medical team, Dave will respond with the serene confidence of a survivor, "No kidding. I had that once." ◆

Appendix

WHERE TO START
ON THE WEB

These Internet sites for prostate cancer are worth checking regularly; they're constantly updated with new information.

www.prostatecancerfoundation.org
Home of the Prostate Cancer Foundation.

www.nlm.nih.gov/medlineplus/prostatecancer.html
This is the website of MedLinePlus, a service of the U.S. Library of Medicine and the National Institutes of Health.

www.cancer.gov/cancertopics/types/prostate
The National Cancer Institute's prostate cancer page.

www.prostate.com/homepage
Though a drug company sponsors the site, it has some interesting features, such as a PSA tracker to help you keep tabs on your tests.

www.cancer.org
The American Cancer Society website.

Index

OTHER BOOKS FROM CLEVELAND CLINIC PRESS

Age Well! A Cleveland Clinic Guide

Arthritis: A Cleveland Clinic Guide

Autopsy – Learning from the Dead: A Cleveland Clinic Guide

Battling the Beast Within: Success in Living with Adversity
    (about multiple sclerosis)

Bladder Cancer: A Cleveland Clinic Guide

Breastless in the City: A Young Woman's Story of Love, Loss,
    and Breast Cancer

Epilepsy – Information for You and Those Who Care About You:
    A Cleveland Clinic Guide

Forever Home
    (a chapter book for young readers)

Getting a Good Night's Sleep: A Cleveland Clinic Guide

The Granny-Nanny: A Guide for Parents and Grandparents
    Who Share Child Care

Headaches: A Cleveland Clinic Handbook

Heart Attack: A Cleveland Clinic Guide

Heroes with a Thousand Faces: True Stories of People with Facial
    Deformities and Their Quest for Acceptance

Lessons Learned: Stroke Recovery from a Caregiver's Perspective

My Grampy Can't Walk
(a children's picture book about multiple sclerosis)

One Stroke, Two Survivors
(the journey of a stroke victim and his wife)

Overcoming Infertility: A Cleveland Clinic Guide

Planting the Roses: A Cancer Survivor's Story
(about esophageal cancer)

Sober Celebrations: Lively Entertaining Without the Spirits
(alcohol-free cooking)

Stop Smoking Now! The Rewarding Journey to a Smoke-Free Life

Tango: Lessons for Life
(a dancing doctor's perspective on healing and life)

Thyroid Disorders: A Cleveland Clinic Guide

To Act As A Unit: The Story of the Cleveland Clinic
(fourth edition)

Transplanting a Face: Notes on a Life in Medicine

Women's Health – Your Body, Your Hormones, Your Choices:
A Cleveland Clinic Guide

Write for Life: Healing Body, Mind, and Spirit Through
Journal Writing

You and Your Cardiologist: A Cleveland Clinic Guide

You CAN Eat That! Awesome Food for Kids with Diabetes

CLEVELAND CLINIC PRESS

Cleveland Clinic Press publishes nonfiction trade books for the medical, health, nutrition, cookbook, and children's markets. It is the mission of the Press to increase the health literacy of the American public and to dispel myths and misinformation about medicine, health care, and treatment. Our authors include leading authorities from Cleveland Clinic as well as a diverse list of experts drawn from medical and health institutions whose research and treatment breakthroughs have helped countless people.

Each Cleveland Clinic Guide provides the health-care consumer with practical and authoritative information. Every book is reviewed for accuracy and timeliness by Cleveland Clinic experts.

www.clevelandclinicpress.org

CLEVELAND CLINIC

Cleveland Clinic, located in Cleveland, Ohio, is a not-for-profit multispecialty academic medical center that integrates clinical and hospital care with research and education. Cleveland Clinic was founded in 1921 by four renowned physicians with a vision of providing outstanding patient care based upon the principles of cooperation, compassion, and innovation. *U.S. News & World Report* consistently names Cleveland Clinic as one of the nation's best hospitals in its annual "America's Best Hospitals" survey. Approximately 1,800 full-time salaried physicians at Cleveland Clinic and Cleveland Clinic Florida represent more than 120 medical specialties and subspecialties. In 2006, patients came for treatment from every state and 100 countries.

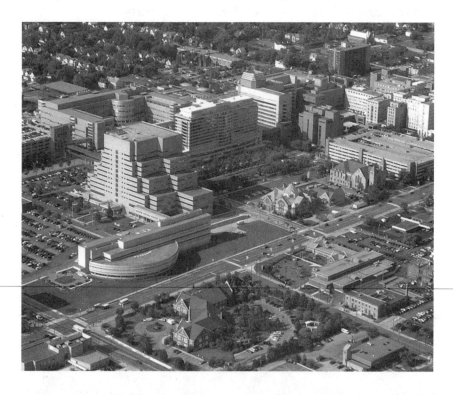